DELMAR'S MATH REVIEW *FOR* HEALTH CARE PROFESSIONALS

THE BASICS OF DECIMALS

Roger W. Ellsbury

Associate Professor
Goodwin College
East Hartford, CT

&

Evening Supervisor
Stone Academy
Waterbury, CT

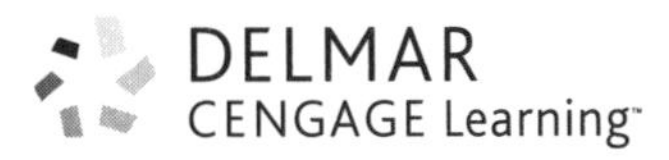

Australia • Brazil • Japan • Korea • Mexico • Singapore • Spain • United Kingdom • United States

DELMAR
CENGAGE Learning™

Delmar's Math Review *for* Health Care Professionals: The Basics of Decimals
Roger W. Ellsbury

Vice President, Career and Professional Editorial: Dave Garza

Director of Learning Solutions: Matthew Kane

Senior Acquisitions Editor: Maureen Rosener

Managing Editor: Marah Bellegarde

Editorial Assistant: Samantha Miller

Vice President, Career and Professional Marketing: Jennifer Baker

Marketing Director: Wendy E. Mapstone

Marketing Manager: Michele McTighe

Marketing Coordinator: Scott A. Chrysler

Production Director: Carolyn Miller

Production Manager: Andrew Crouth

Content Project Management: PreMediaGlobal

Compositor: PreMediaGlobal

Library of Congress Control Number: 2010933017

ISBN-13: 978-1-4390-5837-4

ISBN-10: 1-4390-5837-7

Delmar
5 Maxwell Drive
Clifton Park, NY 12065-2919
USA

Cengage Learning is a leading provider of customized learning solutions with office locations around the globe, including Singapore, the United Kingdom, Australia, Mexico, Brazil, and Japan. Locate your local office at: **international.cengage.com/region**

Cengage Learning products are represented in Canada by Nelson Education, Ltd.

To learn more about Delmar, visit **www.cengage.com/delmar**

Purchase any of our products at your local college store or at our preferred online store **www.cengagebrain.com**

Notice to the Reader

Publisher does not warrant or guarantee any of the products described herein or perform any independent analysis in connection with any of the product information contained herein. Publisher does not assume, and expressly disclaims, any obligation to obtain and include information other than that provided to it by the manufacturer. The reader is expressly warned to consider and adopt all safety precautions that might be indicated by the activities described herein and to avoid all potential hazards. By following the instructions contained herein, the reader willingly assumes all risks in connection with such instructions. The publisher makes no representations or warranties of any kind, including but not limited to, the warranties of fitness for particular purpose or merchantability, nor are any such representations implied with respect to the material set forth herein, and the publisher takes no responsibility with respect to such material. The publisher shall not be liable for any special, consequential, or exemplary damages resulting, in whole or part, from the readers' use of, or reliance upon, this material.

Printed in the United States of America
1 2 3 4 5 14 13 12 11 10

TABLE OF CONTENTS

PREFACE

DELMAR'S MATH REVIEW SERIES FOR HEALTH CARE PROFESSIONALS

This series is designed to assist students who are studying to become healthcare professionals, for those just entering the health care field, and for practicing health care professionals who need to review mathematical concepts. This series assumes that the reader has basic arithmetic skills, particularly a basic understanding of fractional concepts. This series is an ideal companion to a dosage calculation book.

This series is designed as small modules of topic-specific math content. This modular design allows readers the flexibility to choose the areas they want to study. In addition, the books in the series can be used in a classroom or an online class setting, where an instructor presents the material and students practice the concepts presented, or they can be used as supplemental material for readers who want to review the concepts on their own. The explanations and examples are clear enough for readers to follow independently.

The series is designed to enhance the reader's learning experience. The instructional sections are presented in a clear and straightforward manner without distracting graphics or colors. The emphasis is on a basic presentation of the concepts with numerous examples and explanations to illustrate the various applications. The reader has many opportunities to practice the concepts, and answers and explanations to the questions are included so that the reader can immediately check an answer and remediate as necessary.

Series Organization

This four-book module series includes:

Basics of Decimals/ISBN: 1-4390-5837-7

Basics of Fractions/ISBN: 1-4390-5835-0

Basics of Percents/ISBN: 1-4390-5836-9

Basics of Rate, Ratio, and Proportion/ISBN: 1-4390-5838-5

Book Features

Each book contains the following features designed to provide students with straightforward explanations of concepts, examples, practice, and testing situations to check their comprehension of content.

- Each book is organized into small *Sections* to enhance the reading experience.
- *Learning Objectives* found at the beginning of each section focus the reader on the concepts to be covered.
- Multiple *Examples* afford the reader several opportunities to gain an understanding of the content.
- *Exercises,* found after each concept presentation, allow readers to check their comprehension before moving on to new content.
- A *Section Test* is included at the end of each section. Here students assess their understanding of the concepts they studied.
- *Answers* with detailed explanations for all Exercises, all Review Exercises, and the Section Test are included at the end of each section, allowing readers to check their work and remediate as necessary.
- A *Summary* contains all of the important information presented in the book. Readers can review the summary before taking the Cumulative Test. Readers also will find the Summary to be an invaluable reference for future use.
- A *Cumulative Test* allows students to assess their knowledge of all concepts presented in the book. The *Answers* are provided immediately after the test.

ABOUT THE AUTHOR

Roger Ellsbury is a full-time Associate Professor at Goodwin College in East Hartford, Connecticut, where he has been teaching math, English, and computer courses for seven years. His extensive background as an educator included 25 years of public school teaching, after which time he became Senior Facilitator for the Academy of Learning in Waterbury, Connecticut, teaching end-user software to adults.

Continuing his career as an educator, he accepted a position as instructor of Integrated Computer Technology at Stone Academy in Waterbury, where he taught Mathematics for Science and Technology along with various courses in computer technology. Later he taught Medical Terminology, Medical Law and Ethics, Professional Development, Business Communications, English Fundamentals, and Communication Skills for Health Care Professionals. While at Stone Academy, he was promoted to and currently holds the position of Evening Supervisor. In this position, he is responsible for the staff, faculty, and students in the evening programs. He has also conducted in-service training sessions in computer software for the staff and faculty.

After receiving Bachelor of Arts and a Master of Arts degrees at the University of Connecticut, Roger continued his studies at Saint Joseph College in Connecticut. He earned a Certificate of Advanced Graduate Study (CAGS) in special education. In the field of computer technology, he has earned A+, Network+, and Microsoft Office User Specialist (Master Level) certifications. He has also received a Diploma from the Academy of Learning in Computer Software Applications.

ACKNOWLEDGEMENTS

I would like to thank Goodwin College for its support with this project.

I also would like to thank all the people at Delmar, Cengage Learning who have had a hand in this project, especially Maureen Rosener whose vision and understanding has helped turn my idea into reality. Her guidance and suggestions have been invaluable.

I would especially like to thank my wife Linda for her support, tolerance, and patience. Her advice based on years of experience in education and her excellent proofreading abilities have made this project even better.

REVIEWER LIST

Michele Bach, MS
Kansas City Kansas Community College
Kansas City, Kansas

Susan Carlson, MS, RN, CS, NPP
Monroe Community College
Rochester, New York

Irene Coons, MSN, RN, CNE
College of Southern Nevada
Las Vegas, Nevada

Patricia Sunderhaus, MSN Ed, RN
Brown Mackie College
Cincinnati, Ohio

Margie Barondeau Washnok, APRN, MS, DNP
Presentation College
Aberdeen, South Dakota

SECTION **1**

Decimal Concepts

OBJECTIVES

Upon completion of this section, you should be able to:

1. Locate decimal points in numbers when the decimal points are not visible.
2. Determine place value of a specified digit in a decimal number.
3. Read a decimal number properly.
4. Write a decimal number in digits properly.
5. Add necessary zeros to a decimal.
6. Remove unnecessary zeros from a decimal.
7. Compare decimal numbers.
8. Round decimals to a fixed place value.

LOCATING DECIMAL POINTS

The **decimal point** appears just to the right of the units (also called ones) place value and separates the whole number portion from the decimal portion of the number. Every number has a decimal point, yet it may not always be visible. When a number does not have a decimal in it, the decimal point is usually not shown. If the decimal point is not visible, it is located just to the right of the last digit in the number.

Example 1

The decimal point in the number 123 is not visible. Locate the decimal point.

The decimal point is always just to the right of the last digit in the whole number. So the decimal point for 123 is just to the right of the 3.

The answer is 123.

Note: Do not confuse a decimal point with a period that ends a sentence. When a number with a decimal point comes at the end of a sentence, use only one dot, not two. The answer is never "123.."

DETERMINING PLACE VALUE

Compare these two amounts: $543.21 and $123.45. The first amount represents more money. Notice that each amount has a dollar sign, a decimal point, and the same digits 1 through 5, yet the amounts are different because of how the digits are positioned. The position of a digit in relationship to the digits around it is called **place value.**

Study the place value chart in Figure 1–1

← Number gets larger — Number gets smaller →

Whole Numbers								Decimal Numbers					
Millions	Hundred Thousands	Ten Thousands	Thousands	Hundreds	Tens	Units or Ones	Decimal Point	Tenths	Hundredths	Thousandths	Ten-thousandths	Hundred-thousandths	Millionths

Figure 1-1

Some facts about decimals:

- In reading a number, the decimal point is read as *and.* The word *and* is not said anywhere else in the number.
- Numbers to the right of the decimal point are smaller than 1, and numbers to the left of the decimal point are whole numbers.

- Starting from the decimal point and moving to the left in the whole number portion, a comma is used to separate groups of three digits.
- No commas are used to the right of the decimal point.
- All decimal places end with the letters *ths.*
- All of the decimal place values have a corresponding whole number place value.
- There is no corresponding decimal position for the units position.
- The decimal places of ten-thousandths and hundred-thousandths use a hyphen, while ten thousands and hundred thousands places do not.
- If there is no whole number with the decimal, place a zero in the units place.

Example 2

The value of a digit depends on its place in the number. Answer the following questions about place value using the number at the right. The answers follow.

123,456.789

2a. Does this number have two decimal points?

2b. Which digit is in the units place?

2c. Which digit is in the tens place?

2d. Which digit is in the tenths place?

2e. Which digit is in the hundreds place?

2f. Which digit is in the hundredths place?

2g. Which digit is in the thousandths place?

2h. Which digit is in the thousands place?

2i. Which digit is in the ten thousands place?

2j. Which digit is in the hundred thousands place?

Answers to Example 2

2a. No, a number never has two decimal points. In some cases, the second point may be the period that ends a sentence. The decimal point in this number is between the 6 and the 7.

2b. 6 is in the units place. The decimal point is just to its right.

2c. 5 is in the tens place. Locate the decimal point before starting to look for the place value. Do not automatically start with the digit at the far right of the number. If your answer was 8, you did not start at the decimal point.

2d. 7 is in the tenths place. Don't confuse tens and tenths.

2e. 4 is in the hundreds place.

2f. 8 is in the hundredths place.

2g. 9 is in the thousandths place.

2h. 3 is in the thousands place.

2i. 2 is in the ten thousands place.

2j. 1 is in the hundred thousands place.

EXERCISES IN DETERMINING PLACE VALUE

(*Answers are on page 12.*)

Underline the digit in the tenths place value.

1. 12.847 2. 19.2364 3. 0.294 4. 1.058

Underline the digit in the hundredths place value.

5. 612.847 6. 517.264 7. 210.294 8. 192.605

Use the number 50,493.82716 to answer the following questions.

9. Which digit is in the units place value?
10. Which digit is in the tens place value?
11. Which digit is in the tenths place value?
12. Which digit is in the thousands place value?
13. Which digit is in the ten-thousandths place value?
14. Which digit is in the hundredths place value?
15. Which digit is in the hundreds place value?

READING DECIMALS NUMBERS

To read a number that has a decimal in it, first read the whole number part of the number. Be sure to say the grouping name (for example, thousand or million). The decimal point is read as *and.* Next, read the decimal part of the number as if it were a whole number. Then say the name of the place value that is farthest to the right. The number 1.234 would be read as follows:

one and two hundred thirty-four thousandths

Example 3

Read the following decimal numbers. The answers are provided at the right.

3a. 0.3 three tenths

3b. 0.34 thirty-four hundredths

3c. 0.345 three hundred forty-five thousandths

3d. 0.3456 three thousand, four hundred fifty-six ten-thousandths

3e. 0.34567 thirty-four thousand, five hundred sixty-seven hundred-thousandths

3f. 1.028 one and twenty-eight thousandths

3g. 1.0028 one and twenty-eight ten-thousandths

3h. 98,765.4321 ninety-eight thousand, seven hundred sixty-five and four thousand, three hundred twenty-one ten-thousandths

WRITING DECIMAL NUMBERS IN DIGITS

To write a number in digits that has a decimal in it, first write the digits of the whole number portion. Next, place the decimal point. Finally, write the decimal portion of the number. If necessary, use zeros to maintain proper place value.

Remember, when writing decimal numbers in words:

- Use *and* only to represent the decimal point.
- Use a hyphen with the numbers 21 to 99.
- Use commas to separate the groups of numbers in whole numbers.
- Do not use commas to separate groups of numbers in decimals.

Example 4

Write these words as digits. The answers are provided at the right.

4a. three and seven tenths 3.7

4b. two and fifty-four hundredths 2.54

4c. two and fifty-four thousandths 2.054

4d. nine hundredths 0.09

4e. twenty-one and twenty-one thousandths 21.021

4f. one hundred and one hundredth 100.01

4g. seventy-seven thousand and six hundred three ten-thousandths 77,000.0603

IDENTIFYING NECESSARY AND UNNECESSARY ZEROS WITH DECIMALS

> When there is no whole number with a decimal, place a zero in the units place value; this is the leading zero. Its purpose is to help identify the location of the decimal point. There should be only one leading zero.
>
> Zeros may be added to the right of the last nonzero digit of a decimal without changing the value of the number. When the number is given as an answer, these zeros are usually discarded. An exception is made in the case of money. For example, $0.50 is never changed to $0.5.
>
> Calculators generally remove unnecessary zeros at the end of a decimal number. Calculators may also add a zero in the units place when there are no whole numbers.

Example 5

Answer these questions about zeros in decimals. The answers follow.

5a. Which of these numbers is correct: .8, 0.8, or 00.8?

5b. Are these numbers identical in value: 0.5, 0.50, 0.500?

5c. When giving a final answer, which of these is correct: 0.330, .33, 0.33.?

5d. Which of these numbers is correct: 4.790, 04.79, or 4.79?

5e. Which zeros are necessary in this number: 0.60100?

Answers to Example 5

5a. 0.8 is correct. There is no whole number, so a zero is put in the units place. There can be only one leading zero.

5b. Yes, all three numbers are identical in value. Any number of zeros may be added to the right of the last nonzero digit.

5c. 0.33 is correct. It must have a leading zero. Ending zeros are generally removed unless specifically required for the answer.

5d. 4.79 is correct. Ending zeros are removed. Also, because there is a whole number, no leading zero is used.

5e. The leading zero is necessary, and the zero between the 6 and the 1 is necessary for place value. The two ending zeros are not necessary. The number should be 0.601.

COMPARING DECIMALS

> To compare two decimal numbers, first determine the smallest place value of the decimals. Add enough zeros to the other number so that both numbers have the same place values. Then compare the two numbers.

Example 6

Which is larger: 0.27 or 0.3?

Step 1: The smallest place value in these numbers is in the hundredths place.

Step 2: Add one zero to 0.3 so that both numbers have the same place value.

Step 3: Compare 0.27 and 0.30. 0.30 is larger because it has 30 hundredths while the other number only has 27 hundredths.

Example 7

Arrange these numbers from smallest to largest: 0.71, 7.1, 0.071, and 0.701.

Step 1: The smallest place value is the thousandths place.

Step 2: Add zeros so that all numbers have the same place values. This way the numbers can be compared: 0.710, 7.100, 0.071, and 0.701.

Step 3: The smallest number is 0.071 because it has only 71 thousandths. The next smallest number is 0.701 because it has 701 thousandths. The next number is 0.710 because it has 710 thousandths. The largest number is 7.100 because while it only has 100 thousandths, it has 7 units.

Thus: The numbers arranged from smallest to largest are 0.071, 0.701, 0.71, and 7.1. The zeros that were added for comparison are removed when the final answer is given.

EXERCISES IN COMPARING DECIMALS

(*Answers are on page 12.*)

Which of these numbers is larger?

1. 2.04 or 2.4
2. 8.26 or 8.62
3. 0.05 or 0.005
4. 0.403 or 0.43
5. 0.7 or 0.699
6. 3.826539 or 4.3

Arrange these numbers from smallest to largest.

7. 0.05, 0.5, and 5.05
8. 0.73, 0.37, 0.307, and 0.703
9. 0.64, 4.6, 0.46, and 0.406
10. 0.123, 0.1023, 1.23, and 0.1203
11. 0.089, 0.98, 0.908, 0.809, 0.098, and 0.0089
12. 0.5032, 0.2305, 2.305, 0.3502, 0.30502, and 0.5023

ROUNDING DECIMALS TO A FIXED PLACE VALUE

To round to a specific place value:

Step 1: Locate the digit in the specific place value to be rounded. This is the **rounding digit.** You may find that underlining it is helpful.

Step 2: Look at the digit directly to its right. If this digit is 5 or larger, increase the rounding digit by one. If this digit is not 5 or larger, do not change the rounding digit.

Step 3: For places to the right of the decimal point, drop all digits after the rounded digit. If the number represents money, zeros may be added to give two decimal places.

Example 8

Round these numbers to the nearest whole number. The answers are provided at the right.

8a. 14.7 Because the digit in the tenths place is 7 (5 or larger), add 1 to the units place. The answer is 15.

8b. 26.4 Because the digit in the tenths place is 4 (not 5 or larger), the decimals are discarded. The answer is 26.

8c. 9.9 Because the digit in the tenths place is 9 (5 or larger), add 1 to the units place. The answer is 10.

8d. 3.299 Because the digit in the tenths place is 2 (not 5 or larger), the decimals are discarded. The answer is 3. The 9s are ignored.

Example 9

9a. Round 9.7261 to the nearest tenth.

Step 1: Locate the digit in the tenths place. Underlining it is helpful: 9.7261.

Step 2: Because the digit to its right is 2 (not 5 or larger), discard the decimals to the right.

Thus: 9.7261 rounded to the nearest tenth is 9.7.

9b. Round 9.7261 to the nearest hundredth.

Step 1: Locate the digit in the hundredths place. Underlining it is helpful: 9.7261.

Step 2: Because the digit to its right is 6 (5 or larger), add 1 to the hundredths place

Thus: 9.7261 rounded to the nearest hundredth is 9.73.

9c. Round 9.7261 to the nearest thousandth.

Step 1: Locate the digit in the thousandths place. Underlining it is helpful: 9.7261.

Step 2: Because the digit to its right is 1 (not 5 or larger), discard the decimal to the right

Thus: 9.7261 rounded to the nearest thousandth is 9.726.

EXERCISES IN ROUNDING DECIMALS

(*Answers are on page 13.*)

Round these decimals to the nearest tenth.

1. 4.427
2. 4.482
3. 5.939
4. 5.971
5. 0.95

Round these decimals to the nearest hundredth.

6. 3.947
7. 3.944
8. 0.014
9. 0.015
10. 0.07499

Round these decimals to the nearest thousandth.

11. 0.1473
12. 0.1476
13. 0.1005
14. 0.2468
15. 0.9999

EXERCISES IN DECIMAL CONCEPTS

(*Answers are on pages 13–14.*)

Which of these zeros is not necessary in the decimal number? Which of these decimal numbers needs a zero? What should the correct number be?

1. 0.13
2. .130
3. 13.013
4. 0.01300
5. 00.13

Read these decimal numbers aloud.

6. 2.2
7. 0.45
8. 3.007
9. 1.11111
10. 4587.156

Write these decimal numbers in digits.

11. fifteen and two tenths
12. six thousand, seven hundred two and fifty-three thousandths
13. one million, eight hundred thousand twenty-seven and five hundred thirty-one ten-thousandths
14. eighty thousand, four hundred fifteen and sixty-nine thousand, three hundred seventy-seven hundred-thousandths
15. Where is the decimal point in 63 if it is not visible?
16. Which is larger: 0.27 or 0.089?
17. Which is larger: 0.407 or 0.047?
18. Which is the largest: 0.106, 0.061, or 0.16?
19. Which is the largest: 0.3004, 0.034, 0.304, or 0.3?
20. Which is the largest: 0.009, 0.01, 0.00524, or 0.000938?

Arrange these decimal numbers in order from smallest to largest.

21. 0.015, 0.105, 0.0105, and 0.1005
22. 0.38, 0.407, 0.092, 0.0615, and 0.2
23. 0.508, 0.085, 0.85, 0.058, and 0.805

Use the number 98,765.4321 to answer the following questions about place value.

24. Which digit is in the ten thousands place?
25. Which digit is in the tenths place?
26. Which digit is in the hundredths place?

27. Which digit is in the thousandths place?
28. Which digit is in the units place?
29. Which digit is in the hundreds place?
30. Which digit is in the ten-thousandths place?

Round the numbers to the nearest tenth.

31. 0.37
32. 0.73
33. 0.449
34. 0.952
35. 0.09

Round the numbers to the nearest hundredth.

36. 0.874
37. 0.847
38. 0.0192
39. 0.0129
40. 0.999

Round the numbers to the nearest thousandth.

41. 0.1924
42. 0.1925
43. 0.8995
44. 1.0101
45. 0.9999

SECTION TEST: DECIMAL CONCEPTS

(*Answers are on page 14.*)

Why are these decimal numbers not acceptable?

1. 3.86.9
2. 00.4
3. 5.1700
4. Which is larger: 0.062 or 0.26?
5. Arrange these decimal numbers in order from smallest to largest. 0.37, 0.307, 0.73, and 0.703

Use the number 90,817.26354 *to answer the following questions about place value and rounding.*

6. What digit is in the hundredths place?
7. What digit is in the thousands place?
8. What digit is in the ten-thousandths place?
9. What digit is in the tenths place?
10. Round the number to the nearest whole number.
11. Round the number to the nearest thousandth.
12. Round the number to the nearest tenth.
13. Round the number to the nearest hundredth.
14. Write this number in digits: seven thousand and seven hundredths.
15. Write this number in digits: one hundred sixty-seven ten-thousandths.

ANSWERS TO EXERCISES IN DETERMINING PLACE VALUE

(Exercises are on page 4.)

1. 12.847 2. 19.2364 3. 0.294 4. 1.058

5. 612.847 6. 517.264 7. 210.294 8. 192.605

9. 3 is in the units place value.
10. 9 is in the tens place value.
11. 8 is in the tenths place value.
12. 0 is in the thousands place value.
13. 1 is in the ten-thousandths place value.
14. 2 is in the hundredths place value.
15. 4 is in the hundreds place value.

ANSWERS TO EXERCISES IN COMPARING DECIMALS

(Exercises are on page 8.)

1. 2.4. is larger. Compare 2.04 and 2.40.
2. 8.62. is larger. Compare 8.26 and 8.62.
3. 0.05. is larger. Compare 0.050 and 0.005.
4. 0.43. is larger. Compare 0.403 and 0.430.
5. 0.7. is larger. Compare 0.700 and 0.699.
6. 4.3 is larger. Compare 3.826539 and 4.300000.
7. 0.05, 0.5, 5.05
8. 0.307, 0.37, 0.703, 0.73
9. 0.406, 0.46, 0.64, 4.6
10. 0.1023, 0.1203, 0.123, 1.23
11. 0.0089, 0.089, 0.098, 0.809, 0.908, 0.98
12. 0.2305, 0.30502, 0.3502, 0.5023, 0.5032, 2.305

ANSWERS TO EXERCISES IN ROUNDING DECIMALS

(Exercises are on page 9.)

1. 4.4	2. 4.5	3. 5.9	4. 6	5. 1
6. 3.95	7. 3.94	8. 0.01	9. 0.02	10. 0.07
11. 0.147	12. 0.148	13. 0.101	14. 0.247	15. 1

ANSWERS TO EXERCISES IN DECIMAL CONCEPTS

(Exercises are on pages 10–11.)

1. This number is correct. The leading zero is necessary.
2. This number needs a leading zero, but the ending zero is not necessary. The correct number is 0.13.
3. This number is correct. The zero in the tenths place is needed for place value.
4. The leading zero and the zero in the tenths place are needed. The two ending zeros are not necessary. The correct number is 0.013.
5. There should be only one leading zero. The first zero is not necessary. The correct number is 0.13.
6. two and two tenths
7. forty-five hundredths
8. three and seven thousandths
9. one and eleven thousand, one hundred eleven hundred-thousandths
10. four thousand, five hundred eighty-seven and one hundred fifty-six thousandths
11. 15.2
12. 6,702.053
13. 1,800,027.0531
14. 80,415.69377
15. The decimal point is just after the units place: 63.
16. 0.27 is larger. Compare 0.270 and 0.089.
17. 0.407 is larger. Compare 0.407 and 0.047.
18. 0.16 is the largest. Compare 0.106, 0.061, and 0.160.
19. 0.304 is the largest. Compare 0.3004, 0.0340, 0.3040, and 0.3000.
20. 0.01 is the largest. Compare 0.009000, 0.010000, 0.005240, and 0.000938.

21. 0.0105, 0.015, 0.1005, 0.105
22. 0.0615, 0.092, 0.2, 0.38, 0.407
23. 0.058, 0.085, 0.508, 0.805, 0.85
24. 9 is in the ten thousands place.
25. 4 is in the tenths place.
26. 3 is in the hundredths place.
27. 2 is in the thousandths place.
28. 5 is in the units place.
29. 7 is in the hundreds place.
30. 1 is in the ten-thousandths place.

31. 0.4	32. 0.7	33. 0.4	34. 1	35. 0.1
36. 0.87	37. 0.85	38. 0.02	39. 0.01	40. 1
41. 0.192	42. 0.193	43. 0.9	44. 1.01	45. 1

ANSWERS TO SECTION TEST: DECIMAL CONCEPTS

(Section Test is on page 11.)

1. A number cannot have two decimal points.
2. There cannot be two leading zeros.
3. The two zeros at the end of the number are not necessary.
4. 0.26 is larger. Compare 0.062 and 0.260.
5. 0.307, 0.37, 0.703, 0.73
6. 6 is in the hundredths place.
7. 0 is in the thousands place.
8. 5 is in the ten-thousandths place.
9. 2 is in the tenths place.
10. 90,817 is rounded to the nearest whole number.
11. 90,817.264 is rounded to the nearest thousandth.
12. 90,817.3 is rounded to the nearest tenth.
13. 90,817.26 is rounded to the nearest hundredth.
14. 7,000.07
15. 0.0167

SECTION 2

Addition of Decimals

OBJECTIVES

Upon completion of this section, you should be able to:

1. Line up decimal numbers properly for addition.
2. Add decimal numbers correctly without carrying.
3. Add decimal numbers correctly by carrying.
4. Solve application problems using addition.

LINING UP DECIMALS IN ADDITION

The addition of decimals is identical to the addition of whole numbers. Lining up the decimal points ensures that the place values are positioned properly. If a decimal does not appear in a number, the decimal point is immediately after the last digit.

To add the numbers 12.3 and 4.56, the digit 4 is placed beneath the digit 2, not the digit 1. This is because both the 4 and the 2 are in the units position. The decimal points are just to the right of the units position. Once the decimal points are lined up properly, the digits are lined up according to their place values. It is often necessary to add extra zeros to indicate empty place values. This helps keep the numbers lined up and visually assists in addition.

Incorrect:
```
   12.3
+ 4.56
```
Correct:
```
  12.30
+  4.56
```

Example 1

Position these numbers for addition: 12.34 and 67.8. Do not add the numbers.

Step 1:	Write the first number.	12.34
Step 2:	Position the second number so that the decimal points line up.	+ 67.80
Step 3:	Add a zero to 67.8.	

Example 2

Position these numbers for addition: 167.39, 35.1, and 1.94. Do not add the numbers.

Step 1:	Write the first number.	167.39
Step 2:	Position the second number.	35.10
Step 3:	Position the third number. Make sure the decimal points line up.	+ 1.94
Step 4:	Add a zero to 35.1.	

Example 3

Position these numbers for addition: $2.00, $2.20, and $0.22. Do not add the numbers.

Step 1:	Write the first number.	$2.00
Step 2:	Position the second number.	$2.20
Step 3:	Position the third number. Make sure the decimal points line up.	+ $0.22

Example 4

Position these numbers for addition: 1.496, 12.3, and 6.81. Do not add the numbers.

Step 1:	Write the first number.	1.496
Step 2:	Position the second number.	12.3
Step 3:	Position the third number.	+ 6.81
Step 4:	Add two zeros to the second number.	1.496
	Add one zero to the third number.	12.300
		+ 6.810

Note: The zeros that are added help to visually align the decimal place values of the numbers.

Example 5

Position these numbers for addition: 0.41, 0.729, 0.1, and 3. Do not add the numbers.

Step 1:	Write the first number.	0.41
Step 2:	Position the second number.	0.729
Step 3:	Position the third number.	0.1
Step 4:	Position the fourth number.	+ 3.
Step 5:	Add one zero to the first number.	0.410
	Add two zeros to the third number.	0.729
	Add three zeros to the fourth number.	0.100
		+ 3.000

When positioned properly, all of the decimal points in the numbers line up.

EXERCISES IN POSITIONING NUMBERS FOR ADDITION

(*Answers are on page 28.*)

Position these numbers for addition, but do not add.

1. 1.239 and 4.821
2. 24.72 and 3.84
3. 57.92 and 57.4
4. 12.16, 15.423, and 8.6
5. 1.6, 2.09, 5.4, and 0.13
6. 1.5, 0.15, 0.015, and 15

ADDING DECIMALS

When adding numbers with decimals in them, start the addition with the column that has the smallest place value. This is the column at the right. Continue to add columns, moving toward the left until all columns are added. The numbers being added are called **addends,** and the answer is called the **sum.**

Example 6

Add these numbers: 3.21 and 1.42.

Step 1: Position the numbers for addition.

$$\begin{array}{r} 3.21 \\ +\ 1.42 \\ \hline \end{array}$$

Step 2: Add the hundredths place values.

$$\begin{array}{r} 3.21 \\ +\ 1.42 \\ \hline 3 \end{array}$$

Step 3: Add the tenths place values.

$$\begin{array}{r} 3.21 \\ +\ 1.42 \\ \hline 63 \end{array}$$

Step 4: Position the decimal point underneath the other decimal points in the problem.

$$\begin{array}{r} 3.21 \\ +\ 1.42 \\ \hline .63 \end{array}$$

Step 5: Add the units place values.

$$\begin{array}{r} 3.21 \\ +\ 1.42 \\ \hline 4.63 \end{array}$$

Thus: $3.21 + 1.42 = 4.63$

CARRYING IN ADDITION

When the sum of the digits for a place value is larger than 9, part of the number is carried to the next place value.

For example, $5 + 8 = 13$. For the number 13, the 1 represents a ten because it is in the tens place value and the 3 represents 3 units ($13 = 10 + 3$). The digit 3 remains in the units place number, and the digit 1 is carried to the tens place.

Example 7

Add these numbers: 2.8 and 1.4.

Step 1: Position the numbers for addition.

$$\begin{array}{r} 2.8 \\ +\ 1.4 \\ \hline \end{array}$$

Step 2: Add the 8 + 4 in the tenths column to get 12. Place 2 in the tenths column and carry the 1 to the units column.

$$\begin{array}{r} {}^{1} \\ 2.8 \\ +\ 1.4 \\ \hline 2 \end{array}$$

Step 3: Position the decimal point underneath the other decimal points in the problem.

$$\begin{array}{r} {}^{1} \\ 2.8 \\ +\ 1.4 \\ \hline .2 \end{array}$$

Step 4: Add 1 + 2 + 1 in the units column to get 4.

$$\begin{array}{r} {}^{1} \\ 2.8 \\ +\ 1.4 \\ \hline 4.2 \end{array}$$

Thus: 2.8 + 1.4 = 4.2

Example 8

Add these numbers: 4.78 and 1.35.

Step 1: Position the numbers for addition.

$$\begin{array}{r} 4.78 \\ +\ 1.35 \\ \hline \end{array}$$

Step 2: Add the 8 + 5 in the hundredths column to get 13. Place 3 in the hundredths column and carry the 1 to the tenths column.

$$\begin{array}{r} {}^{1} \\ 4.78 \\ +\ 1.35 \\ \hline 3 \end{array}$$

Step 3: Add the 1 + 7 + 3 in the tenths column to get 11. Place 1 in the tenths column and carry the 1 to the units column.

$$\begin{array}{r} {}^{1\ 1} \\ 4.78 \\ +\ 1.35 \\ \hline 13 \end{array}$$

Step 3: Position the decimal point underneath the other decimal points in the problem.

$$\begin{array}{r} {}^{1\ 1} \\ 4.78 \\ +\ 1.35 \\ \hline .13 \end{array}$$

Step 4: Add 1 + 4 + 1 in the units column to get 6.

$$\begin{array}{r} {}^{1\ 1} \\ 4.78 \\ +\ 1.35 \\ \hline 6.13 \end{array}$$

Thus: 4.78 + 1.35 = 6.13

Example 9

Add these numbers: 58.74, 7.8, and 6.396.

Step 1: Position the numbers for addition.

$$\begin{array}{r} 58.74 \\ 7.8 \\ +\ 6.396 \\ \hline \end{array}$$

Step 2: Add zeros where necessary.

$$\begin{array}{r} 58.740 \\ 7.800 \\ +\ 6.396 \\ \hline \end{array}$$

Step 3: Add the thousandths column.

$$\begin{array}{r} 58.740 \\ 7.800 \\ +\ 6.396 \\ \hline 6 \end{array}$$

Step 4: Add the hundredths column: 4 + 9 = 13. Place the 3 in the hundredths column and carry the 1 to the tenths column.

$$\begin{array}{r} {\scriptstyle 1} \\ 58.740 \\ 7.800 \\ +\ 6.396 \\ \hline 36 \end{array}$$

Step 5: Add the tenths column: 1 + 7 + 8 + 3 = 19. Place 9 in the tenths column and carry 1 to the units column.

$$\begin{array}{r} {\scriptstyle 1\ 1} \\ 58.740 \\ 7.800 \\ +\ 6.396 \\ \hline 936 \end{array}$$

Step 6: Position the decimal point underneath the other decimal points in the problem.

$$\begin{array}{r} {\scriptstyle 1\ 1} \\ 58.740 \\ 7.800 \\ +\ 6.396 \\ \hline .936 \end{array}$$

Step 7: Add the units column: 1 + 8 + 7 + 6 = 22. Place 2 in the units column and carry 2 to the tens column.

$$\begin{array}{r} {\scriptstyle 2\ 1\ 1} \\ 58.740 \\ 7.800 \\ +\ 6.396 \\ \hline 2.936 \end{array}$$

Step 8: Add the tens column: 2 + 5 = 7.

$$\begin{array}{r} {\scriptstyle 2\ 1\ 1} \\ 58.740 \\ 7.800 \\ +\ 6.396 \\ \hline 72.936 \end{array}$$

Thus: 58.74 + 7.8 + 6.396 = 72.936

EXERCISES WITH CARRYING IN ADDITION

(*Answers are on page 28.*)

Add the following numbers. Carry when necessary.

1. $\begin{array}{r} 8.7 \\ +\ 6.9 \\ \hline \end{array}$

2. $\begin{array}{r} 0.67 \\ +\ 0.96 \\ \hline \end{array}$

3. $\begin{array}{r} 5.48 \\ 6.54 \\ +\ 0.90 \\ \hline \end{array}$

4. $\begin{array}{r} 4.753 \\ 7.126 \\ +\ 1.489 \\ \hline \end{array}$

5. $\begin{array}{r} 21.49 \\ 5.78 \\ +\ 16.84 \\ \hline \end{array}$

6. $\begin{array}{r} 9.999 \\ 0.909 \\ +\ 9.090 \\ \hline \end{array}$

7. $\begin{array}{r} 0.009 \\ 0.098 \\ 0.842 \\ +\ 0.759 \\ \hline \end{array}$

8. $\begin{array}{r} 8.493 \\ 92.617 \\ 9.785 \\ +\ 0.215 \\ \hline \end{array}$

SOLVING ADDITION APPLICATIONS

Use addition to answer questions that ask for the total—or how much something is all together. For the addition process, smaller amounts are combined to make a larger amount.

Steps for Solving an Application Problem

Step 1: Read the problem carefully. Pay close attention to the numbers in the problem.

Step 2: Read the question carefully. What exactly is it looking for? What label will be used in the answer?

Step 3: Eliminate any unnecessary information.

Step 4: Draw a diagram if it is helpful.

Step 5: Decide how to solve the problem. Some problems may require more than one step.

Step 6: Round the numbers to the highest place value and estimate the answer.

Step 7: Calculate the final answer and compare it with the estimate.

Step 8: Include the label in the answer.

Example 10

A vitamin pill contains 0.009 gram of iron. Seven pills are left in the bottle. A supplemental iron pill contains 0.075 gram of iron. How many grams of iron would a patient consume if he took both pills?

Step 1: The two numbers are 0.009 gram of iron and 0.075 gram of iron.

Step 2: The question is asking how many grams of iron these two pills contain.

Step 3: The unnecessary information is the number of pills left in the bottle.

Step 4: Figure 2-1 shows one possible diagram.

0.009 gram	0.075 gram

Figure 2-1

Step 5: The numbers should be added together to get the total number of grams of iron.

Step 6: Estimating to the nearest hundredth of a gram, 0.009 gram becomes 0.01 gram and 0.075 gram becomes 0.08 gram.

Step 7: The estimated answer is $0.01 + 0.08 = 0.09$ gram.

Step 8: Calculate the actual answer to be 0.084.

This answer is close to the estimate of 0.09.

$$\begin{array}{r} 0.009 \text{ gram} \\ +\ 0.075 \text{ gram} \\ \hline 0.084 \text{ gram} \end{array}$$

Thus: The patient would consume 0.084 gram of iron if he took both pills.

Example 11

A nurse monitored the formula consumption of an infant over a 12-hour period. The infant drank 3.2 oz, 2.7 oz, and 3.45 oz. How many ounces of formula did the infant drink?

Step 1: The numbers for the ounces of formula are 3.2, 2.7, and 3.45.

Step 2: The question asks how many ounces of formula the infant drank.

Step 3: The unnecessary information is the 12-hour time period.

Step 4: Figure 2-2 shows one possible diagram.

3.2 oz	2.7 oz	3.45 oz

Figure 2-2

Step 5: The numbers should be added together to get the total number of ounces of formula.

Step 6: Estimating to the nearest ounce, 3.2 oz becomes 3 oz, 2.7 oz becomes 3 oz, and 3.45 oz becomes 3 oz.

Step 7: The estimated answer is 3 oz + 3 oz + 3 oz = 9 oz.

Step 8: Set up the addition problem and add zeros where necessary. Calculate the actual answer to be 9.35 oz, which is close to the estimated answer of 9 oz.

$$\begin{array}{r} 3.20 \text{ oz} \\ 2.70 \text{ oz} \\ +\ 3.45 \text{ oz} \\ \hline 9.35 \text{ oz} \end{array}$$

Thus: The infant drank 9.35 oz of formula.

EXERCISES IN SOLVING ADDITION APPLICATIONS

(Answers are on pages 29–30.)

Use addition to solve these problems.

1. A mother gave birth to triplets: Ava was 43.27 cm long, Daphne was 42.9 cm long, and Cleopatra was 44.64 cm long. Arrange the babies from shortest to tallest. What was the total length of the three babies?

2. A patient received a dose of medication with every meal. She received 2.5 oz with breakfast, 2.5 oz with lunch, and 2.5 oz with supper. How much medication did the patient receive?

3. A patient received a series of injections of medication: 1.7 mL, 2.3 mL, and 2.1 mL. What was the total amount of milliliters the patient received?

4. A patient received a bill for the following: $65.37 for IV tubing, $13.09 for a catheter, and $15.96 for a dressing change kit. What was the patient's total bill?

5. A patient receives 2.1 grams of a mineral in his normal vitamin pill. A nurse supplements this with a tablet containing 4.5 grams of the same mineral. The nurse also calculates that the patient's breakfast will supply him with 3.5 grams of the mineral. How many grams of the mineral has the patient consumed?

6. A patient received the following bills for medication: $71.31, $11.99, $42.10, and 52.24. What was the patient's total bill for the medication?

7. An outpatient weighed 85.4 kg in January. In February, the patient gained 1.8 kg. In March, the patient gained 2.3 kg. How much did the patient weigh in March?

8. Three open bottles of the same cough syrup are in a medicine cabinet. One bottle contains 2.5 fl oz, another contains 1.25 fl oz, and the third contains 3.1 fl oz. How much cough syrup do these bottles contain?

9. A nurse's supper in the hospital cafeteria consisted of $4.99 for a garden salad, $3.89 for a bowl of soup, $1.69 for a cup of coffee, and $1.99 for a package of cookies. How much did the nurse's supper cost?

AVOIDING COMMON MISTAKES IN ADDING DECIMALS

Here are some common mistakes people make when adding decimal numbers:

- Lining up the place values of the numbers improperly
- Using sloppy handwriting or sloppy positioning of the numbers
- Copying the numbers incorrectly
- Carrying improperly
- Using incorrect math facts

SECTION TEST: ADDITION OF DECIMALS

(Answers are on pages 30–31.)

Solve these problems using addition.

1. Add 2.3, 4.05, and 1.23.

2. Add 0.023, 0.014, and 0.062.

3. Add 1.58, 15.8, and 0.158.

4. Add 2, 2.05, 2.005, and 2.5.

5. Add 12.59, 0.3879, and 8.965.

6. Add 0.45, 0.447, and 0.103.

7. A patient's fluid intake for one day was 4.75 oz, 8.5 oz, 5.25 oz, 6.4 oz, and 4.6 oz. What was the patient's total fluid intake for the day?

8. A cold sufferer bought cold medication tablets for $15.99, cough syrup for $4.99, and a box of facial tissues for $2.69. What was the total cost?

9. One sandwich contained 0.36 oz of ham, 0.33 oz of Swiss cheese, 0.27 oz of turkey, and 0.22 oz of roast beef. How many ounces of meat were in the sandwich?

ANSWERS TO EXERCISES IN POSITIONING NUMBERS FOR ADDITION

(Exercises are on page 17.)

1. $$\begin{array}{r} 1.239 \\ \underline{+\ 4.821} \end{array}$$

2. $$\begin{array}{r} 24.72 \\ \underline{+\ 3.84} \end{array}$$

3. $$\begin{array}{r} 57.92 \\ \underline{+\ 57.40} \end{array}$$

4. $$\begin{array}{r} 12.160 \\ 15.423 \\ \underline{+\ 8.600} \end{array}$$

5. $$\begin{array}{r} 1.60 \\ 2.09 \\ 5.40 \\ \underline{+\ 0.13} \end{array}$$

6. $$\begin{array}{r} 1.500 \\ 0.150 \\ 0.015 \\ \underline{+\ 15.000} \end{array}$$

ANSWERS TO EXERCISES WITH CARRYING IN ADDITION

(Exercises are on page 21.)

1. $$\begin{array}{r} {\scriptstyle 1\ \ \ } \\ 8.7 \\ \underline{+\ 6.9} \\ 15.6 \end{array}$$

2. $$\begin{array}{r} {\scriptstyle 1\ 1\ \ } \\ 0.67 \\ \underline{+\ 0.96} \\ 1.63 \end{array}$$

3. $$\begin{array}{r} {\scriptstyle 1\ 1\ \ } \\ 5.48 \\ 6.54 \\ \underline{+\ 0.90} \\ 12.92 \end{array}$$

4. $$\begin{array}{r} {\scriptstyle 1\ 11\ } \\ 4.753 \\ 7.126 \\ \underline{+\ 1.489} \\ 13.368 \end{array}$$

5. $$\begin{array}{r} {\scriptstyle 1\ 2\ 2\ } \\ 21.49 \\ 5.78 \\ \underline{+\ 16.84} \\ 44.11 \end{array}$$

6. $$\begin{array}{r} {\scriptstyle 1\ 11\ } \\ 9.999 \\ 0.909 \\ \underline{+\ 9.090} \\ 19.998 \end{array}$$

7. $$\begin{array}{r} {\scriptstyle 1\ 22\ } \\ 0.009 \\ 0.098 \\ 0.842 \\ \underline{+\ 0.759} \\ 1.708 \end{array}$$

8. $$\begin{array}{r} {\scriptstyle 22\ 22\ } \\ 8.493 \\ 92.617 \\ 9.785 \\ \underline{+\ 0.215} \\ 111.110 \end{array}$$

Note: For problem 8, the last zero is dropped. The answer is 111.11.

ANSWERS TO EXERCISES IN SOLVING ADDITION APPLICATIONS

(Exercises are on pages 24–25.)

1. From shortest to tallest, the babies are Daphne at 42.90 cm long, Ava at 43.27 cm long, and Cleopatra at 44.64 cm long.

   Add the three lengths to get the total length of the babies.

$$\begin{array}{r} {\scriptstyle 1\,1\;\;1}\phantom{.00\text{ cm}} \\ 42.90\text{ cm} \\ 43.27\text{ cm} \\ +\ 44.64\text{ cm} \\ \hline 130.81\text{ cm} \end{array}$$

   The total length of the three babies was 130.81 cm.

2. Add the three doses of medication to get the total amount of medication the patient received with her meals.

$$\begin{array}{r} {\scriptstyle 1}\phantom{.5\text{ oz}} \\ 2.5\text{ oz} \\ 2.5\text{ oz} \\ +\ 2.5\text{ oz} \\ \hline 7.5\text{ oz} \end{array}$$

   The patient received 7.5 oz of medication.

3. Add the three injections of medication to get the total amount of milliliters of medication the patient received.

$$\begin{array}{r} {\scriptstyle 1}\phantom{.7\text{ mL}} \\ 1.7\text{ mL} \\ 2.3\text{ mL} \\ +\ 2.1\text{ mL} \\ \hline 6.1\text{ mL} \end{array}$$

   The patient received 6.1 mL of medication.

4. Add the cost of the three items to get the total bill.

$$\begin{array}{r} {\scriptstyle 1\,1\;\;2} \\ \$65.37 \\ \$13.09 \\ +\ \$15.96 \\ \hline \$94.42 \end{array}$$

   The patient's total bill was $94.42.

5. Add the three amounts to get the total grams of the mineral.

$$\begin{array}{r} {\scriptstyle 1}\phantom{.1\text{ grams}} \\ 2.1\text{ grams} \\ 4.5\text{ grams} \\ +\ 3.5\text{ grams} \\ \hline 10.1\text{ grams} \end{array}$$

   The patient has consumed 10.1 grams of the mineral.

6. Add the four bills for medication to get the total amount of the bill.

$$\begin{array}{r} {\scriptstyle 1\;\;1} \\ \$71.31 \\ \$11.99 \\ \$42.10 \\ +\ \$52.24 \\ \hline \$177.64 \end{array}$$

   The patient's total bill for medication was $177.64.

7. Add the three weights to get the total amount the patient weighed in March.

```
    1
 85.4 kg
  1.8 kg
+ 2.3 kg
--------
 89.5 kg
```

The patient weighed 89.5 kg in March.

8. Add the three amounts of the cough syrup to get the total amount the bottles contain.

```
  2.50 fl oz
  1.25 fl oz
+ 3.10 fl oz
------------
  6.85 fl oz
```

The bottles contain 6.85 fl oz.

9. Add the four costs of the items the nurse bought to get the total amount of the bill for her supper.

```
   3 3
  $4.99
  $3.89
  $1.69
+ $1.99
-------
 $12.56
```

The nurse's supper cost $12.56.

ANSWERS TO SECTION TEST: ADDITION OF DECIMALS

(Section Test is on pages 26–27.)

```
1.   2.30      2.   0.023      3.   1 1
     4.05           0.014           1.580
   + 1.23         + 0.062          15.800
   ------         -------         + 0.158
     7.58           0.099         -------
                                   17.538

4.   2.000     5.  11 21       6.  1 11
     2.050         12.5900          0.450
     2.005          0.3879          0.447
   + 2.500        + 8.9650        + 0.103
   -------        --------        -------
     8.555         21.9429          1.000
```

Note: For problem 6, the zeroes are dropped. The answer is 1.

7. Add the five numbers to calculate the patient's total fluid intake.

$$\begin{array}{r} {\scriptstyle 2\ 1} \\ 4.75 \text{ oz} \\ 8.50 \text{ oz} \\ 5.25 \text{ oz} \\ 6.40 \text{ oz} \\ +\ 4.60 \text{ oz} \\ \hline 29.50 \text{ oz} \end{array}$$

   The patient's total fluid intake for the day was 29.5 oz.

8. Add the cost of the three items to get the total cost for the cold sufferer.

$$\begin{array}{r} {\scriptstyle 1\ 2\ 2} \\ \$15.99 \\ \$4.99 \\ +\ \$2.69 \\ \hline \$23.67 \end{array}$$

   The total cost was $23.67.

9. The question asks for the ounces of *meat* in the sandwich. Because Swiss cheese is not meat, do not include it in the calculation. Add the three amounts to get the total amount of meat in the sandwich.

$$\begin{array}{r} {\scriptstyle 1} \\ 0.36 \text{ oz} \\ 0.27 \text{ oz} \\ +\ 0.22 \text{ oz} \\ \hline 0.85 \text{ oz} \end{array}$$

   There was 0.85 oz of meat in the sandwich.

SECTION **3**

Subtraction of Decimals

OBJECTIVES

Upon completion of this section, you should be able to:

1. Explain the connection between addition and subtraction.
2. Set up a subtraction problem properly.
3. Subtract without borrowing.
4. Check a subtraction problem using addition.
5. Subtract with borrowing.
6. Work with zeros when borrowing.
7. Solve application problems using subtraction.

SUBTRACTION CONCEPTS

Subtraction is often called the opposite of addition. When one number is added to another, the answer is the **sum.** When one of the numbers is subtracted from the sum, the other number is the **difference.**

Example 1

Observe the similarity of this sample addition problem with its opposite subtraction problem.

A sample addition problem:

$$\begin{array}{rl} 0.2 & \text{(the first number)} \\ \underline{+\ 0.4} & \text{(the second number)} \\ 0.6 & \text{(their sum)} \end{array}$$

The sample subtraction problem using the same numbers:

$$\begin{array}{rl} 0.6 & \text{(the previous sum)} \\ \underline{-\ 0.2} & \text{(the first number)} \\ 0.4 & \text{(the second number)} \end{array}$$

This is an alternative subtraction problem using the same numbers.

$$\begin{array}{rl} 0.6 & \text{(the previous sum)} \\ \underline{-\ 0.4} & \text{(the second number)} \\ 0.2 & \text{(the first number)} \end{array}$$

SETTING UP A SUBTRACTION PROBLEM

The same rules used for addition apply to subtraction: line up the decimal points in the numbers and add zeros if necessary. Sometimes the way a problem is worded can be confusing. It is important to know which number is the starting point (the top number in a subtraction problem). If the problem is worded *subtract 12 from 36,* 36 is the starting number. Thus, it is on top. On the other hand, if the problem is worded *40 minus 18,* 40 is the starting number.

Example 2

Set up these subtraction problems, but do not solve them.

2a. *1.09 minus 0.31*

$$\begin{array}{r} 1.09 \\ -\ 0.31 \\ \hline \end{array}$$

Because 0.31 is being taken away from 1.09, 1.09 is the top number.

2b. *Subtract 16.91 from 20*

$$\begin{array}{r} 20.00 \\ -\ 16.91 \\ \hline \end{array}$$

Because 16.91 is being subtracted from 20, 20 is the top number. A decimal point is added after the 20 to align the numbers. Two zeros are added to 20 to make it 20.00.

2c. *Subtract 8.4 from 9.03.*

$$\begin{array}{r} 9.03 \\ -\ 8.40 \\ \hline \end{array}$$

Because 8.4 is subtracted from 9.03, 9.03 is the top number. A zero must be added after the 4 in the second number so that the numbers line up properly.

2d. *2.047 minus 1.89.*

$$\begin{array}{r} 2.047 \\ -\ 1.890 \\ \hline \end{array}$$

Because 1.89 is being subtracted from 2.047, 2.047 is the top number. A zero must be added after the 9 in the second number.

EXERCISES IN SETTING UP SUBTRACTION PROBLEMS

(*Answers are on page 50.*)

Set up these subtraction problems, but do not solve them.

1. Subtract 0.9 from 2.3.

2. 0.3 minus 0.03

3. Take 0.82 from 8.2.

4. Subtract 0.01 from 0.1.

SUBTRACTING WITHOUT BORROWING

> As in addition, begin subtracting with the smallest place value. This is the place value farthest to the right. Continue subtracting each place value in order from right to left.

Example 3

The following subtraction example is completed in stages to show the process.

$$\begin{array}{r} 5.82 \\ -\ 3.21 \\ \hline 1 \end{array}$$

Start subtraction with the smallest place value. In this problem, it is the hundredths place value: $2 - 1 = 1$. Place the 1 in the hundredths column.

$$\begin{array}{r} 5.82 \\ -\ 3.21 \\ \hline 61 \end{array}$$

Subtract the next place value to the left which is the tenths: $8 - 2 = 6$. Place the 6 in the tenths column.

$$\begin{array}{r} 5.82 \\ -\ 3.21 \\ \hline .61 \end{array}$$

Position the decimal point underneath the other decimal points.

$$\begin{array}{r} 5.82 \\ -\ 3.21 \\ \hline 2.61 \end{array}$$

Subtract the last column: $5 - 3 = 2$. Place 2 in the units column.

Thus: $5.82 - 3.21 = 2.61$

CHECKING A SUBTRACTION PROBLEM

> Because addition is the opposite of subtraction, addition is used to check the answer to a subtraction problem. Add the answer to the number being subtracted; the result will be the top number.

Example 4

Subtract 0.12 from 5.69 and use addition to check the problem.

$$\begin{array}{r} 5.69 \\ -\ 0.12 \\ \hline \end{array}$$

First, set up the problem correctly. Because 0.12 is being subtracted from 5.69, 5.69 is the top number.

$$\begin{array}{r} 5.69 \\ -\ 0.12 \\ \hline 5.57 \end{array}$$

Begin subtracting from the farthest place value to the right. Continue subtracting the rest of the place values in order.

Make sure the decimal point in the answer lines up with the other decimal points in the problem.

Thus: When 0.12 is subtracted from 5.69, the answer is 5.57.

Check the answer by using addition. Add the answer (5.57) and the number being subtracted (0.12). The result should be the top number in the subtraction problem (5.69).

$$\begin{array}{r} 5.57 \\ +\ 0.12 \\ \hline 5.69 \end{array}$$

Add the hundredths column: $7 + 2 = 9$ hundredths. Add the tenths column: $5 + 1 = 6$ tenths. Position the decimal point. Add the units column: $5 + 0 = 5$. The answer checks.

EXERCISES IN SUBTRACTION WITHOUT BORROWING

(*Answers are on page 50.*)

Use subtraction to calculate the answers to these problems. Use addition to check your work.

1. $\begin{array}{r} 8.96 \\ -\ 3.62 \\ \hline \end{array}$

2. $\begin{array}{r} 78.5 \\ -\ 44.2 \\ \hline \end{array}$

3. $\begin{array}{r} 9.475 \\ -\ 3.174 \\ \hline \end{array}$

4. $\begin{array}{r} 29.685 \\ -\ 18.351 \\ \hline \end{array}$

SUBTRACTING WITH BORROWING

In addition, when an amount is larger than 9, part of it is **carried** to the next place value. In subtraction, there is an opposite process called **borrowing.** An amount is removed from a larger place value, and its equivalent is added to the smaller place value.

Sometimes it is necessary to borrow more than once in a problem. This is especially true when zeros are in the top number.

Example 5

The following is an example of the concept of borrowing.

Consider the number 31. The 3 is in the tens place value, so it represents 30. The 1 is in the units place value, so it represents 1. The number 31 represents 30 + 1.

$$\begin{array}{r} 31 \\ -\ 5 \\ \hline \end{array}$$

In this problem, 5 units cannot be subtracted from 1 unit, so it is necessary to borrow from the tens column.

As stated earlier, the 3 in 31 is in the tens column, and it represents a value of 30. In borrowing from the tens column, the 3 tens will become 2 tens. The 1 that is borrowed (which represents 10) is added to the units place value (1) to get 11. So through borrowing, 31 is changed to 20 and 11.

(When added together, 20 + 11 = 31.)

So $\begin{array}{r} 31 \\ -\ 5 \\ \hline \end{array}$ becomes $\begin{array}{r} {\scriptstyle 2\ 11} \\ \not{3}\not{1} \\ -\ 5 \\ \hline 26 \end{array}$ Now 5 can be subtracted from 11 to get 6, and the 2 is brought down to get 26.

Thus: 31 − 5 = 26.

Check the answer by using addition.

$$\begin{array}{r} {\scriptstyle 1\ \ } \\ 26 \\ +\ 5 \\ \hline 31 \end{array}$$

Add the units column: 6 + 5 = 11. Because 11 units is equivalent to 1 ten and 1 unit, 1 ten is carried to the tens column. Add the tens column: 1 + 2 = 3.

The answer checks.

Example 6

The borrowing process is used in this subtraction problem.

$$\begin{array}{r} 4.0 \\ -\ 1.7 \\ \hline \end{array}$$

Because 7 tenths cannot be subtracted from 0 tenths, 1 unit from the next larger place value is "borrowed." The number 4 units and 0 tenths is changed to 3 units and 10 tenths.

$$\begin{array}{r} {\scriptstyle 3\ \ 10} \\ \not{4}.\not{0} \\ -\ 1.7 \\ \hline 2.3 \end{array}$$

Now 7 tenths can be subtracted from 10 tenths to give an answer of 3 tenths. The decimal point is positioned. 1 unit is subtracted from 3 units to give 2 units.

Thus: $4.0 - 1.7 = 2.3$

Check the answer by using addition.

$$\begin{array}{r} {\scriptstyle 1} \\ 1.7 \\ +\ 2.3 \\ \hline 4.0 \end{array}$$

Add the tenths column: $7 + 3 = 10$ tenths. Because 10 tenths is equivalent to 1 unit, 1 unit is carried to the units column. Position the decimal point. Add the units column: $1 + 1 + 2 = 4$ units. The answer checks.

Example 7

This is another example of the borrowing process.

$$\begin{array}{r} 7.5 \\ -\ 2.9 \\ \hline \end{array}$$

9 tenths cannot be subtracted from 5 tenths, so 1 unit is borrowed from the 7 units. The 7 units becomes 6 units, and the 1 unit that is borrowed is changed to 10 tenths. The 10 tenths is added to the existing 5 tenths to give 15 tenths. 7 units and 5 tenths is changed to 6 units and 15 tenths.

$$\begin{array}{r} {\scriptstyle 6\ \ 15} \\ \not{7}.\not{5} \\ -\ 2.9 \\ \hline 4.6 \end{array}$$

9 tenths is subtracted from 15 tenths to give 6 tenths. The decimal point is positioned under the other decimal points. 2 units is subtracted from 6 units to give 4 units.

Thus: $7.5 - 2.9 = 4.6$.

Check the answer by using addition.

$$\begin{array}{r} {\scriptstyle 1} \\ 2.9 \\ +\ 4.6 \\ \hline 7.5 \end{array}$$

Add the tenths column: $9 + 6 = 15$ tenths. Because 15 tenths is equivalent to 1 unit and 5 tenths, 1 unit is carried to the units column. Position the decimal point. Add the units column: $1 + 2 + 4 = 7$. The answer checks.

Example 8

In this problem, it is necessary to borrow more than once.

$$\begin{array}{r} {\scriptstyle 5\ 12} \\ 8.\cancel{6}\cancel{2} \\ -\ 3.65 \\ \hline \end{array}$$

5 hundredths cannot be subtracted from 2 hundredths, so 1 tenth is borrowed from the tenths column and is added to the hundredths column.

$$\begin{array}{r} {\scriptstyle 5\ 12} \\ 8.\cancel{6}\cancel{2} \\ -\ 3.65 \\ \hline 7 \end{array}$$

Subtract the hundredths column: 12 − 5 = 7. The 6 tenths cannot be subtracted from the 5 tenths, so 1 unit is borrowed from the units column.

$$\begin{array}{r} {\scriptstyle 15\ \ \ } \\ {\scriptstyle 7\ \cancel{5}\ 12} \\ \cancel{8}.\cancel{6}\cancel{2} \\ -\ 3.65 \\ \hline 4.97 \end{array}$$

Subtract the tenths column: 15 − 6 = 9. Subtract the units column: 7 − 3 = 4.

Thus: 8.62 − 3.65 = 4.97

Check the answer by using addition.

$$\begin{array}{r} {\scriptstyle 1\ \ } \\ 4.97 \\ +\ 3.65 \\ \hline 2 \end{array}$$

Add the hundredths column: 7 + 5 = 12 hundredths. Because 12 hundredths is equivalent to 1 tenth and 2 hundredths, 1 tenth is carried to the tenths column.

$$\begin{array}{r} {\scriptstyle 1\ 1\ \ } \\ 4.97 \\ +\ 3.65 \\ \hline 62 \end{array}$$

Add the tenths column: 1 + 9 + 6 = 16 tenths. Because 16 tenths is equivalent to 1 unit and 6 tenths, 1 unit is carried to the units column.

$$\begin{array}{r} {\scriptstyle 1\ 1\ \ } \\ 4.97 \\ +\ 3.65 \\ \hline 8.62 \end{array}$$

Position the decimal point. Add the units: 1 + 4 + 3 = 8 units. The answer checks.

EXERCISES IN SUBTRACTING WITH BORROWING

(*Answers are on page 50.*)

Use subtraction and borrowing to calculate the answers to these problems. Check your answers by using addition.

1. $\begin{array}{r} 24.16 \\ -\ 6.25 \\ \hline \end{array}$
2. $\begin{array}{r} 3.91 \\ -\ 0.95 \\ \hline \end{array}$
3. $\begin{array}{r} 119.1 \\ -\ 89.3 \\ \hline \end{array}$
4. $\begin{array}{r} 3.528 \\ -\ 0.749 \\ \hline \end{array}$

WORKING WITH ZEROS WHEN BORROWING

> When borrowing, if a zero is in the next column, it is necessary to borrow from the next nonzero column. When there is more than one zero, continue to the next nonzero column to borrow.

Example 9

Observe what happens when borrowing with zero in a number.

$$\begin{array}{r} 0.102 \\ -\ 0.085 \\ \hline \end{array}$$

5 cannot be subtracted from 2, so it is necessary to borrow. Because the next place value is zero, it is necessary to borrow from the next nonzero column.

$$\begin{array}{r} {\scriptstyle 0\ 10} \\ 0.\not{1}\not{0}2 \\ -\ 0.085 \\ \hline \end{array}$$

Borrowing 1 from the tenth column leaves zero in the tenths column and 10 in the hundredths column. Once this is done, it is possible to borrow from the hundredths place.

$$\begin{array}{r} {\scriptstyle 9} \\ {\scriptstyle 0\ \not{10}\ 12} \\ 0.\not{1}\not{0}\not{2} \\ -\ 0.085 \\ \hline \end{array}$$

Borrowing 1 from the hundredths place, leaves 9 hundredths and 10 thousandths. Thus, 0.102 has become 0.09 and 12 thousandths.

$$\begin{array}{r} {\scriptstyle 9} \\ {\scriptstyle 0\ \not{10}\ 12} \\ 0.\not{1}\not{0}\not{2} \\ -\ 0.085 \\ \hline 0.017 \end{array}$$

Now 5 thousandths can be subtracted from 12 thousandths. Next, 8 hundredths can be subtracted from 9 hundredths. Finally, 0 tenths can be subtracted from 0 tenths to give an answer of 0.017.

Thus: $0.102 - 0.085 = 0.017$

Check the answer by using addition.

$$\begin{array}{r} {\scriptstyle 1\ 1} \\ 0.017 \\ +\ 0.085 \\ \hline 0.102 \end{array}$$

Add the thousandths column: $7 + 5 = 12$ thousandths. 1 is carried to the hundredths place. Add the hundredths column: $1 + 1 + 8 = 10$ hundredths. 1 is carried to the tenths column. Position the decimal point and supply a leading zero. The answer checks.

Example 10

Observe what happens when borrowing with more than one zero in the number. Subtract 0.248 from 1.

$$\begin{array}{r} 1.000 \\ -\,0.248 \\ \hline \end{array}$$

Three zeros need to be added after the decimal point to line up the place values. 8 cannot be subtracted from 0, so it is necessary to borrow. The first nonzero digit to the left is in the units place value.

$$\begin{array}{l} {\scriptstyle 0\ \ 10} \\ \cancel{1}.\cancel{0}00 \end{array}$$

Borrowing 1 from the units place leaves 0 units and 10 tenths.

$$\begin{array}{l} {\scriptstyle \ \ \ \ \ 9} \\ {\scriptstyle 0\ \cancel{10}\ 10} \\ \cancel{1}.\cancel{0}\cancel{0}0 \end{array}$$

Borrowing 1 from the tenths place leaves 9 tenths and 10 hundredths.

$$\begin{array}{l} {\scriptstyle \ \ \ \ \ 9\ \ \ 9} \\ {\scriptstyle 0\ \cancel{10}\ \cancel{10}\ 10} \\ \cancel{1}.\cancel{0}\cancel{0}\cancel{0} \end{array}$$

Borrowing 1 from the hundredths place leaves 9 hundredths and 10 thousandths.

$$\begin{array}{r} {\scriptstyle 9\ \ \ 9\ \ \ \ } \\ {\scriptstyle 0\ \cancel{10}\ \cancel{10}\ 10} \\ \cancel{1}.\cancel{0}\cancel{0}\cancel{0} \\ -\,0.2\,4\,8 \\ \hline 0.7\,5\,2 \end{array}$$

Now 8 thousands can be subtracted from 10 thousandths.
Next, 4 hundredths can be subtracted from 9 hundredths.
Finally, 2 tenths can be subtracted from 9 tenths.

Thus: $1 - 0.248 = 0.752$

Check the answer by using addition.

$$\begin{array}{r} {\scriptstyle 1\ \ 1\ 1\ \ } \\ \cancel{0}.\cancel{7}\cancel{5}2 \\ +\,0.248 \\ \hline 1.000 \\ 1.000 = 1 \end{array}$$

Add the thousandths column: $2 + 8 = 10$ thousandths. Because 10 thousandths is equivalent to 1 hundredth, 1 is carried to the hundredths column. Add the hundredths column: $1 + 5 + 4 = 10$ hundredths. Because 10 hundredths is equivalent to 1 tenth, 1 is carried to the tenths column. Add the tenths column: $1 + 7 + 2 = 10$ tenths. Because 10 tenths is equivalent to 1 unit, 1 is carried to the units column. Position the decimal point. Add the units column: $1 + 0 + 0 = 1$. The zeros after the decimal point are dropped.

The answer is 1. The answer checks.

EXERCISES IN SUBTRACTING WITH BORROWING AND ZEROS

(*Answers are on page 50.*)

Use subtraction with borrowing to calculate the answers to these problems. Check your answers by using addition.

1. $\begin{array}{r} 5.0604 \\ -\ 0.3827 \\ \hline \end{array}$

2. $\begin{array}{r} 8.0802 \\ -\ 3.2323 \\ \hline \end{array}$

3. $\begin{array}{r} 20.00 \\ -\ 18.99 \\ \hline \end{array}$

4. $\begin{array}{r} 1.502 \\ -\ 0.403 \\ \hline \end{array}$

5. $\begin{array}{r} 0.6000 \\ -\ 0.0802 \\ \hline \end{array}$

6. $\begin{array}{r} 20.40 \\ -\ 8.06 \\ \hline \end{array}$

7. $\begin{array}{r} 10.101 \\ -\ 9.192 \\ \hline \end{array}$

8. $\begin{array}{r} 5.000 \\ -\ 0.024 \\ \hline \end{array}$

9. $\begin{array}{r} 1.000 \\ -\ 0.592 \\ \hline \end{array}$

SOLVING SUBTRACTION APPLICATIONS

Use subtraction to answer questions that ask for the difference between two numbers. The following key words may indicate the need to subtract: *how much greater than; how much less than; how much of an increase or decrease; how many more;* and *how much farther, bigger, smaller, or heavier.* For the subtraction process, a smaller amount is generally removed from an overall amount.

Use the same process for solving a subtraction application problem that is used for solving addition problems.

Steps for Solving an Application Problem

Step 1: Read the problem carefully. Pay close attention to the numbers in the problem.

Step 2: Read the question carefully. What exactly is it looking for? What label will be used in the answer?

Step 3: Eliminate any unnecessary information.

Step 4: Draw a diagram if it is helpful.

Step 5: Decide how to solve the problem. Some problems may require more than one step.

Step 6: Round the numbers to the highest place value and estimate the answer.

Step 7: Calculate the final answer and compare it with the estimate.

Step 8: Include the label in the answer.

Example 11

3.2 fl oz have been removed from a bottle containing 8 fl oz. How many fluid ounces remain in the bottle?

Step 1: The numbers in the problem are 3.2 fl oz and 8 fl oz.

Step 2: The question asks how many fluid ounces are left in a bottle after 3.2 fluid ounces have been removed. This indicates a subtraction problem.

Step 3: Figure 3-1 shows a possible diagram.

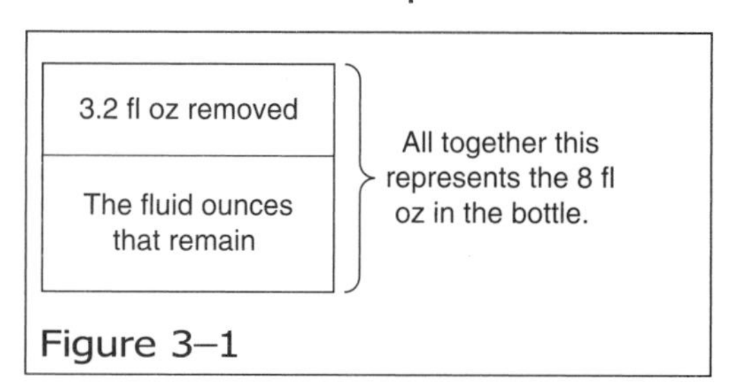

Figure 3–1

Step 4: The 3.2 fl oz removed from the bottle must be subtracted from the total of 8 fl oz to find the number of fluid ounces that remain.

Step 5: Rounding both numbers to the highest place value, which is the units place, 3.2 fl oz becomes 3 fl oz, and 8 fl oz remains 8 fl oz.

Step 6: The estimated answer is 8 fl oz − 3 fl oz = 5 fl oz.

Step 7: Position the numbers for subtraction by lining up the decimal points. Add a zero to the right of 8. Calculate the exact answer to be 4.8 fl oz. That is close to the estimated answer of 5 fl oz.

$$\begin{array}{r} {}^{7}\,{}^{10} \\ \cancel{8}.\cancel{0} \text{ fl oz} \\ -\ 3.2 \text{ fl oz} \\ \hline 4.8 \text{ fl oz} \end{array}$$

Thus: After 3.2 fl oz have been removed from the bottle, 4.8 fl oz remain.

Check the answer by using addition.

$$\begin{array}{r} {}^{1}\quad\quad\quad \\ 3.2 \text{ fl oz} \\ +\ 4.8 \text{ fl oz} \\ \hline 8.0 \text{ fl oz} \end{array}$$

Add the tenths column: 2 + 8 = 10 tenths. Because 10 tenths is equivalent to 1 unit, 1 is carried to the units place. Position the decimal point. Add the units column: 1 + 3 + 4 = 8. The zero to the right of the decimal point is removed.
The answer checks.

Example 12

Normal body temperature is 98.6°F. A patient has a body temperature of 99.6°F. How much higher than normal is the patient's body temperature?

Step 1: The numbers in the problem are 98.6°F and 99.6°F.

Step 2: The question is asking how much higher the patient's body temperature is than the normal body temperature. This indicates a subtraction problem.

Step 3: Figure 3-2 shows a possible diagram.

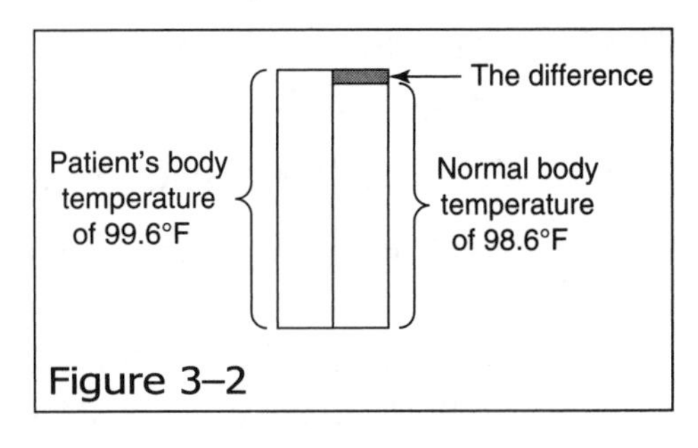

Figure 3–2

Step 4: The normal 98.6°F needs to be subtracted from the patient's 99.6°F to find out how much higher the patient's body temperature is.

Step 5: Rounding both numbers to the highest place value, which is the tens place, 98.6°F becomes 100°F and 99.6°F becomes 100°F.

Step 6: The estimated answer is 100°F − 100°F = 0°F.

Step 7: Position the numbers for subtraction by lining up the decimal points. Calculate the exact answer to be 1.0°F. When reporting the answer, drop the zero. Considering that the overall temperature is nearly 100°F, 1°F is close to the estimated answer of 0°F.

$$\begin{array}{r} 99.6°F \\ -\ 98.6°F \\ \hline 1.0°F \end{array}$$

Thus: The patient's body temperature is 1°F higher than normal.

Check the answer by using addition.

$$\begin{array}{r} 98.6°F \\ +\ 1.0°F \\ \hline 99.6°F \end{array}$$

Add the tenths column: 6 + 0 = 6 tenths. Position the decimal point. Add the units column: 8 + 1 = 9 units. Add the tens column: 9 = 9 tens. The answer checks.

Example 13

An elderly patient weighed 64.4 kg. She lost 2.7 kg. What is her weight now?

Step 1: The numbers in the problem are 64.4 kg and 2.7 kg.

Step 2: The question is asking for the patient's weight now. This indicates a subtraction problem. Subtracting the kilograms lost from the original kilograms will give how much the patient weighs now.

Step 3: Rounding to the highest place value, which is the tens, 64.4 kg becomes 64 kg and 2.7 kg becomes 0 kg.

Step 4: Estimate the answer as 64 kg − 0 kg = 64 kg.

Step 5: Position the numbers for subtraction by lining up the decimal points. Calculate the exact answer to be 61.7 kg. 61.7 kg is close to the estimate of 64 kg. (The difference between the estimate and the exact answer is a result of how much the numbers were rounded.)

```
   3 14
  64.4 kg
−  2.7 kg
  61.7 kg
```

Thus: The patient's weight now is 61.7 kg.

Check the answer by using addition.

```
    1
   2.7 kg
+ 61.7 kg
  64.4 kg
```

Add the tenths column: 7 + 7 = 14 tenths. Because 14 tenths is equivalent to 1 unit and 4 tenths, carry 1 to the units column. Position the decimal point. Add the units column: 1 + 2 + 1 = 4 units. Add the tens column: 6 = 6 tens. The answer checks.

EXERCISES IN SUBTRACTION APPLICATIONS

(*Answers are on page 51.*)

Solve these application problems using subtraction.

1. A medical supply company sells a walker for $27.99 which it bought wholesale for $16.24. What was the company's profit?

2. Disposable medicine spoons sell for $0.125 each. Each spoon costs $0.0875 to make. How much profit is made on one spoon?

3. A study by a major university found that the average life expectancy for females is 79.4 years and for males is 72.7 years. According to this study, how much longer does the average female expect to live than the average male?

4. A patient should have received 2.25 g of medication. The nurse mistakenly gave her 22.5 g instead. How much more medication did the patient receive?

5. A name brand cold remedy sells for $24.99, while a drugstore sells a generic brand under its own name for $16.28. If the sizes of the bottles are the same, how much more expensive is the name brand?

6. A patient weighed 185.4 lb before getting sick. After a lengthy recovery period, the patient weighed 167.6 lb. How much weight did the patient lose?

EXERCISES IN MIXED APPLICATIONS

(Answers are on page 52.)

Solve these application problems using addition and/or subtraction.

1. A bottle of cough syrup holds 7.5 fl oz. If 1.5 fl oz is given to a cold sufferer, how much cough syrup is left?

2. A medical supply company buys bedpans wholesale for $5.73 each. If the company wants to make $1.65 profit per bedpan, what must it charge for each bedpan?

3. In a weight loss program, a participant weighed 214.5 lb before starting and 208.7 lb one month later. How much did the participant lose?

4. A patient weighing 83.9 kg gains 4.53 kg in a one-month period. What is the patient's new weight?

5. A nurse ran 1.6 km on Monday, 2.1 km on Wednesday, and 1.8 km on Friday. The previous week the nurse had run 7.2 km. How much farther did the nurse run last week?

6. A patient's bill totaled $78.64. The patient's medical plan paid $45 for the procedure. The patient had to make a $20 co-pay. Because of an agreement with the insurance company, the doctor could not collect on the remainder of the bill. What was the amount the doctor could not collect?

SECTION TEST: SUBTRACTING DECIMALS

(*Answers are on page 53.*)

Subtract these decimal numbers, borrowing when necessary. Check your answers by using addition.

1. Subtract 0.34 from 0.87.

2. What is 1.96 minus 0.55?

3. Subtract 49¢ from $1.

4. $\begin{array}{r} 5.999 \\ -\ 0.256 \\ \hline \end{array}$

5. $\begin{array}{r} 8.94 \\ -\ 3.57 \\ \hline \end{array}$

6. $\begin{array}{r} 67.54 \\ -\ 48.25 \\ \hline \end{array}$

7. $\begin{array}{r} 32.89 \\ -\ 23.98 \\ \hline \end{array}$

8. $\begin{array}{r} 0.1010 \\ -\ 0.0101 \\ \hline \end{array}$

9. $\begin{array}{r} 5.05 \\ -\ 4.15 \\ \hline \end{array}$

10. $\begin{array}{r} 20.5 \\ -\ 0.6 \\ \hline \end{array}$

11. $\begin{array}{r} 1.776 \\ -\ 0.789 \\ \hline \end{array}$

12. $\begin{array}{r} \$100.00 \\ -\ \$37.59 \\ \hline \end{array}$

13. A bottle contains a total of 8 fl oz of cough medication. If a patient receives a 2.5 fl oz dosage, how much medication is left in the bottle?

14. A woman was brought to the emergency room with a body temperature was 95.3°F. If normal body temperature is 98.6°F, how far below normal was her temperature?

15. A vial holds a total of 6.5 mL of medication. If an injection of 1.6 mL is withdrawn from the vial, how much medication is left in the vial?

ANSWERS TO EXERCISES IN SETTING UP SUBTRACTION PROBLEMS

(*Exercises are on page 35.*)

1. $\begin{array}{r} 2.3 \\ -\ 0.9 \\ \hline \end{array}$

2. $\begin{array}{r} 0.30 \\ -\ 0.03 \\ \hline \end{array}$

3. $\begin{array}{r} 8.20 \\ -\ 0.82 \\ \hline \end{array}$

4. $\begin{array}{r} 0.10 \\ -\ 0.01 \\ \hline \end{array}$

ANSWERS TO EXERCISES IN SUBTRACTING WITHOUT BORROWING

(*Exercises are on page 37.*)

1. $\begin{array}{r} 8.96 \\ -\ 3.62 \\ \hline 5.34 \end{array}$

2. $\begin{array}{r} 78.5 \\ -\ 44.2 \\ \hline 34.3 \end{array}$

3. $\begin{array}{r} 9.475 \\ -\ 3.174 \\ \hline 6.301 \end{array}$

4. $\begin{array}{r} 29.685 \\ -\ 18.351 \\ \hline 11.334 \end{array}$

ANSWERS TO EXERCISES IN SUBTRACTING WITH BORROWING

(*Exercises are on page 40.*)

1. $\begin{array}{r} 24.16 \\ -\ 6.25 \\ \hline 17.91 \end{array}$

2. $\begin{array}{r} 3.91 \\ -\ 0.95 \\ \hline 2.96 \end{array}$

3. $\begin{array}{r} 119.1 \\ -\ 89.3 \\ \hline 29.8 \end{array}$

4. $\begin{array}{r} 3.528 \\ -\ 0.749 \\ \hline 2.779 \end{array}$

ANSWERS TO EXERCISES IN SUBTRACTING WITH BORROWING AND ZEROS

(*Exercises are on page 43.*)

1. $\begin{array}{r} 5.0604 \\ -\ 0.3827 \\ \hline 4.6777 \end{array}$

2. $\begin{array}{r} 8.0802 \\ -\ 3.2323 \\ \hline 4.8479 \end{array}$

3. $\begin{array}{r} 20.00 \\ -\ 18.99 \\ \hline 1.01 \end{array}$

4. $\begin{array}{r} 1.502 \\ -\ 0.403 \\ \hline 1.099 \end{array}$

5. $\begin{array}{r} 0.6000 \\ -\ 0.0802 \\ \hline 0.5198 \end{array}$

6. $\begin{array}{r} 20.40 \\ -\ 8.06 \\ \hline 12.34 \end{array}$

7. $\begin{array}{r} 10.101 \\ -\ 9.192 \\ \hline 0.909 \end{array}$

8. $\begin{array}{r} 5.000 \\ -\ 0.024 \\ \hline 4.976 \end{array}$

9. $\begin{array}{r} 1.000 \\ -\ 0.592 \\ \hline 0.408 \end{array}$

ANSWERS TO EXERCISES IN SUBTRACTION APPLICATIONS

(Exercises are on page 47.)

1. $\begin{array}{r} \$27.99 \\ -\ \underline{\$16.24} \\ \$11.75 \end{array}$

   Calculate the company's profit by subtracting the wholesale price from the retail price of the walker.

   The company's profit was $11.75.

2. $\begin{array}{r} \$0.1250 \\ -\ \underline{\$0.0875} \\ \$0.0375 \end{array}$

   Subtract the cost of a medicine spoon from its selling price to find the profit on one spoon.

   The profit on one spoon is $0.0375.

3. $\begin{array}{r} 79.4\text{ yr} \\ -\ \underline{72.7\text{ yr}} \\ 6.7\text{ yr} \end{array}$

   Subtract the average life expectancy for males from the average life expectancy for females to find out how much longer females are expected to live.

   The answer is 6.7 years.

4. $\begin{array}{r} 22.50\text{ g} \\ -\ \underline{2.25\text{ g}} \\ 20.25\text{ g} \end{array}$

   Subtract what the patient should have received from what the patient was given to find the difference in medication.

   The patient received 20.25 g more medication than she should have.

5. $\begin{array}{r} \$24.99 \\ -\ \underline{\$16.28} \\ \$8.71 \end{array}$

   Subtract the price of the generic brand from the name brand to find how much more expensive the name brand is.

   The name brand is $8.71 more expensive.

6. $\begin{array}{r} 185.4\text{ lb} \\ -\ \underline{167.6\text{ lb}} \\ 17.8\text{ lb} \end{array}$

   Subtract the weight of the patient after recovering from the patient's weight before getting sick to find how much weight the patient lost. The patient lost 17.8 pounds.

ANSWERS TO EXERCISES IN MIXED APPLICATIONS

(Exercises are on page 48.)

1.
$$\begin{array}{r} 7.5 \text{ fl oz} \\ -\ 1.5 \text{ fl oz} \\ \hline 6.0 \text{ fl oz} \end{array}$$

This is a subtraction problem. Subtract the amount given to the cold sufferer from the original amount in the bottle to find the amount of cough syrup left in the bottle.

There are 6 fl oz left.

2.
$$\begin{array}{r} \$5.73 \\ +\ \$1.65 \\ \hline \$7.38 \end{array}$$

This is an addition problem. Add the desired profit to the cost of each bedpan to find the selling price.

The company must charge $7.38 for each bedpan.

3.
$$\begin{array}{r} 214.5 \text{ lb} \\ -\ 208.7 \text{ lb} \\ \hline 5.8 \text{ lb} \end{array}$$

This is a subtraction problem. Subtract the amount weighed after one month from the original amount weighed to find the amount lost. The participant lost 5.8 lb in one month.

4.
$$\begin{array}{r} 83.90 \text{ kg} \\ +\ 4.53 \text{ kg} \\ \hline 88.43 \text{ kg} \end{array}$$

This is an addition problem. Add the weight gained to the original weight to find the new weight.

The patient's new weight is 88.43 kg.

5.
$$\begin{array}{r} 1.6 \text{ km} \\ 2.1 \text{ km} \\ +\ 1.8 \text{ km} \\ \hline 5.5 \text{ km} \end{array}$$

This is a multistep problem. First, add the distances for this week (Monday, Wednesday, and Friday). Next, subtract this number from the distance run last week to find how much farther the nurse ran last week.

$$\begin{array}{r} 7.2 \text{ km} \\ -\ 5.5 \text{ km} \\ \hline 1.7 \text{ km} \end{array}$$

Last week the nurse ran 7.2 km.
This week the nurse ran 5.5 km.
The nurse ran 1.7 km farther last week.

6.
$$\begin{array}{r} \$45 \\ +\ \$20 \\ \hline \$65 \end{array}$$

Add the insurance payment and the patient's co-pay to find how much the doctor was paid.

The doctor was paid $65.

$$\begin{array}{r} \$78.64 \\ -\ \$65.00 \\ \hline \$13.64 \end{array}$$

Subtract what the doctor was paid from the original bill to find how much the doctor could not collect.

The doctor could not collect $13.64.

ANSWERS TO SECTION TEST: SUBTRACTING DECIMALS

(Section Test is on page 49.)

1. $\begin{array}{r} 0.87 \\ -\,0.34 \\ \hline 0.53 \end{array}$

2. $\begin{array}{r} 1.96 \\ -\,0.55 \\ \hline 1.41 \end{array}$

3. $\begin{array}{r} \$1.00 \\ -\,\$0.49 \\ \hline \$0.51 \end{array}$

4. $\begin{array}{r} 5.999 \\ -\,0.256 \\ \hline 5.743 \end{array}$

5. $\begin{array}{r} 8.94 \\ -\,3.57 \\ \hline 5.37 \end{array}$

6. $\begin{array}{r} 67.54 \\ -\,48.25 \\ \hline 19.29 \end{array}$

7. $\begin{array}{r} 32.89 \\ -\,23.98 \\ \hline 8.91 \end{array}$

8. $\begin{array}{r} 0.1010 \\ -\,0.0101 \\ \hline 0.0909 \end{array}$

9. $\begin{array}{r} 5.05 \\ -\,4.15 \\ \hline 0.90 \end{array}$

10. $\begin{array}{r} 20.5 \\ -\,0.6 \\ \hline 19.9 \end{array}$

11. $\begin{array}{r} 1.776 \\ -\,0.789 \\ \hline 0.987 \end{array}$

12. $\begin{array}{r} \$100.00 \\ -\,\$37.59 \\ \hline \$62.41 \end{array}$

13. $\begin{array}{r} 8.0 \text{ fl oz} \\ -\,2.5 \text{ fl oz} \\ \hline 5.5 \text{ fl oz} \end{array}$

Subtract the dosage the patient received from the contents of the bottle to find the amount of medication left.
There are 5.5 fl oz left in the bottle.

14. $\begin{array}{r} 98.6°\text{F} \\ -\,95.3°\text{F} \\ \hline 3.3°\text{F} \end{array}$

Subtract the woman's temperature from normal body temperature to find how far below normal her temperature was. The woman's temperature was 3.3°F below normal.

15. $\begin{array}{r} 6.5 \text{ mL} \\ -\,1.6 \text{ mL} \\ \hline 4.9 \text{ mL} \end{array}$

Subtract the injection amount from the vial's contents to find how much medication is left in the vial.
There are 4.875 mL of medication left in the vial.

SECTION 4

Multiplication of Decimals

OBJECTIVES

Upon completion of this section, you should be able to:

1. Position numbers for multiplication.
2. Position the decimal point in the answer.
3. Multiply a one-digit number times another number.
4. Multiply a multi-digit number times another number.
5. Use the carrying process in multiplication.
6. Work with zeros in multiplication.
7. Solve application problems using multiplication.

MULTIPLICATION CONCEPTS

When multiplying numbers, it does not matter which number is on the top and which is on the bottom. The answer will be the same. Generally, the number with the fewest digits is on the bottom to make the multiplication easier.

The major difference between the process of multiplication of decimals and the process of addition and subtraction of decimals is that in multiplication, the decimal points are *not* lined up. The numbers to be multiplied are written without regard to their place value. After the numbers are multiplied, the decimal point is positioned in the answer.

Example 1

Position these numbers properly for multiplication: multiply 6.853 by 19.4. Do not multiply.

$$\begin{array}{r} 6.853 \\ \times\ 19.4 \\ \hline \end{array}$$

Position one number on the top. Place the second number under the first number so that both are aligned at the right. Decimal points are ignored for now.

Example 2

Position these numbers properly for multiplication: multiply 97.3 by 0.642. Do not multiply.

$$\begin{array}{r} 97.3 \\ \times\ 0.642 \\ \hline \end{array}$$

The first number is written. The second number is aligned directly beneath the number above. Decimal points are ignored for now.

POSITIONING THE DECIMAL POINT IN AN ANSWER

> The position of the decimal point in an answer is determined once the numbers are multiplied. First, count the number of places to the right of the decimal points in both numbers. Second, starting from the far right place value, move the decimal point in the answer the same number of places to the left. If no decimal appears in a number, the decimal is assumed to be just to the right of the last digit.

Example 3

This multiplication problem is almost complete. All it needs is to have the decimal point positioned properly. Notice how the position of the decimal point is located in the answer.

$$\begin{array}{r} 41.3 \\ \times\ 0.21 \\ \hline 413 \\ 8260 \\ \hline 8673 \end{array}$$

There is one decimal place in the first number.
There are two decimal places in the second number.
There are a total of three decimal places in the problem.
Starting from the far right in the answer, move the decimal point three places to the left to position it between the 8 and the 6: 8.673.

Thus, $41.3 \times 0.21 = 8.673$

Note: In the second answer line, a zero is used to position 826 properly. See page 59 for a more detailed explanation of this.

Example 4

Position the decimal point in the answer to this problem.

1.23	There are two decimal places in the first number.
× 4.53	There are two decimal places in the second number.
369	There are a total of four decimal places in this problem.
6150	Starting from the far right in the answer, move the decimal point four
49200	places to the left to position it between the two 5s: 5.5719.
55719	

Thus, 1.23 × 4.53 = 5.5719

Note: See page 59 for an explanation of the extra zeros in 6150 and 49200.

Example 5

Position the decimal point in the answer to this problem.

3.527	There are three decimal places in this number.
× 0.11	There are two decimal places in this number.
3527	There are a total of five decimal places in the problem.
35270	Move the decimal point five places to the left in the answer to position
38797	it just to the left of the 3. A zero must be added to include a leading
	zero: 0.38797.

Thus, 3.527 × 0.11 = 0.38797

Note: See page 59 for an explanation of the extra zeros in 35270.

If there are not enough decimal places in the answer to reposition the decimal point, additional zeros may need to be added. If the decimal point appears before the first nonzero digit, be sure to add a leading zero.

Example 6

Position the decimal point in the answer to this problem.

0.00032	There are five decimal places in this number.
× 0.011	There are three decimal places in this number.
32	There are a total of eight decimal places in the problem.
320	Starting from the far right in the answer, move the decimal point eight
352	places to the left. Five zeros must be added to the left of the number
	to position the decimal point properly.
	A leading zero must also be added. The number is 0.00000352.

Thus, 0.00032 × 0.11 = 0.00000352

Note: See the page 59 for an explanation of the extra zero in 320.

MULTIPLYING A ONE-DIGIT NUMBER TIMES ANOTHER NUMBER

To multiply one digit times another number, position the numbers for multiplication. Then multiply the bottom number times each of the digits in the top number from right to left. Record the answer below the line. Finally, position the decimal point properly.

Example 7

First, position the numbers for multiplication. Next, multiply the numbers correctly. Finally, place the decimal point in the answer. Multiply 0.413 by 0.2.

$$\begin{array}{r} 0.413 \\ \times\ 0.2 \\ \hline 6 \end{array}$$

The numbers are positioned for multiplication without regard to their decimal points. Multiply the bottom digit of 2 times the first digit of 3 in the top number to get 6. Place the 6 under the 2.

$$\begin{array}{r} 0.413 \\ \times\ 0.2 \\ \hline 26 \end{array}$$

Now multiply the 2 times the second digit of 1 in the top number to get 2. Place 2 to the left of 6 in the answer.

$$\begin{array}{r} 0.413 \\ \times\ 0.2 \\ \hline 826 \end{array}$$

Now multiply the 2 times the third digit of 4 in the top number to get 8. Place 8 to the left of 2 in the answer. No further multiplication is needed because the only digit left is a leading zero. Also, no multiplication is needed with the leading zero next to the 2 in the second number.

$$\begin{array}{r} 0.413 \\ \times\ 0.2 \\ \hline 0.0826 \end{array}$$

Next, count the number of decimal places in the multiplication problem. There are a total of four. Move the decimal point in the answer four places to the left starting with the 6. Add a zero before the 8 to position the decimal point properly. Also add a leading zero before the decimal point: 0.0826.

Thus, $0.413 \times 0.2 = 0.0826$

MULTIPLYING A MULTI-DIGIT NUMBER TIMES ANOTHER NUMBER

To multiply a multi-digit number times another number, position the numbers for multiplication. Then multiply the first digit in the second number times all of the digits in the first number and record the answer below the line. This is the first line of the answer.

Next, multiply by the second digit in the second number. Because the second digit is actually in the tens place, put a zero in the units place in the second line of the answer. This preserves proper place value. Then multiply the second digit times all of the numbers in the top number and record the answer on the second answer line.

If there is a third digit to be multiplied, place two zeros on the third answer line because the third digit is actually in the hundreds place. Continue multiplying as before. (Subsequent digits are handled in the same manner.)

When all of the digits have been multiplied, add all of the lines of the answer to get the final answer. Finally, position the decimal point properly.

Example 8

First, position the numbers for multiplication. Next, multiply the numbers. Finally, place the decimal point in the answer. Multiply 43.13 by 1.2. (This problem is completed step-by-step so that you can see the entire process.)

43.13 $\times$ 1.2 6	The numbers are positioned for multiplication without regard to their decimal points. Multiply the bottom digit of 2 times the first digit of 3 in the top number to get 6.
43.13 $\times$ 1.2 26	Now multiply the 2 times the second digit of 1 in the top number to get 2. Place 2 to the left of 6 in the answer.
43.13 $\times$ 1.2 626	Now multiply the 2 times the third digit of 3 in the top number to get 6. Place 6 to the left of 2 in the answer.
43.13 $\times$ 1.2 8626	Finally, multiply the 2 times the fourth digit of 4 in the top number to get 8. Place 8 to the left of 6 in the answer. This completes the multiplication of the first digit (2).
43.13 $\times$ 1.2 8626 0	The next step is to multiply by the second digit in the bottom number. Because this digit is in the tens place, place a zero under the 6 in the first line of the answer to indicate no units.
43.13 $\times$ 1.2 8626 30	Now multiply the 1 in the bottom number times the first digit of 3 in the top number to get 3. Place 3 next to the 0 in the second line of the answer.
43.13 $\times$ 1.2 8626 43130	In the same manner, multiply the 1 in the bottom number times the rest of the digits in the top number. Place each answer in the appropriate place in the second line of the answer.
43.13 $\times$ 1.2 8626 43130 51756	Now add the numbers in both lines of the answer. 8626 + 43130 = 51756. The next step is to position the decimal point. There are two decimal places in the top number and one decimal place in bottom number for a total of three decimal places. Move the the decimal point three places to the left starting with the 6 to position it between the 1 and the 7: 51.756.

Thus, $43.13 \times 1.2 = 51.756$

Example 9

First, position the numbers for multiplication. Next, multiply the numbers correctly. Finally, place the decimal point in the answer. Multiply 0.0134 by 0.222.

$$\begin{array}{r} 0.0134 \\ \times\ 0.222 \\ \hline 268 \end{array}$$

The numbers are positioned without regard to their decimal points. Multiply the first bottom digit of 2 times the top number to get 268. Ignore the leading zeros. This is the first line of the answer.

$$\begin{array}{r} 0.0134 \\ \times\ 0.222 \\ \hline 268 \\ 2680 \end{array}$$

Place a zero in the units position of the second line of the answer because the number multiplied is in the tens place. Then multiply the second bottom digit of 2 times the top number to get 268. Place this in the second line of the answer next to the zero.

$$\begin{array}{r} 0.0134 \\ \times\ 0.222 \\ \hline 268 \\ 2680 \\ 26800 \\ \hline 29748 \end{array}$$

Place zeros in the tens and units positions of the third line of the answer because the number being multiplied is in the hundreds place. Multiply the third bottom digit of 2 times the top number to get 268. Place this in the third line of the answer next to the two zeros. Add the three lines of the answer to get 29748.

There are four decimal places in the first number and three decimal places in the second number for a total of seven. Move the decimal point seven places to the left starting with the 8, but notice that the number 29748 has only five digits. Two zeros must be added to place the decimal point properly. A third zero must be added for the leading zero: 0.0029748.

Thus, $0.0134 \times 0.222 = 0.0029748$

Example 10

Multiply 0.0432 by 0.000012.

$$\begin{array}{r} 0.0432 \\ \times\ 0.000012 \\ \hline 864 \end{array}$$

Position the numbers for multiplication. Multiply the first digit of 2 times the top number to get 864. Ignore the leading zeros. Place this number in the first line of the answer.

$$\begin{array}{r} 0.0432 \\ \times\ 0.000012 \\ \hline 864 \\ \underline{4320} \\ 5184 \end{array}$$

Put a zero in the units place of the second answer line because the multiplying number is in the tens place. Now multiply the second digit of 1 times the top number to to get 432. Place this number next to the zero in the second line of the answer. Add both answer lines to get 5184.

There are four decimal places in the first number and six decimal places in the second number for a total of ten. The decimal point must be moved ten places to the left in the answer starting with the 4; however, the answer has only four digits. Six zeros must be added to position the decimal point properly. A seventh zero must be added to include a leading zero: 0.0000005184.

Thus, $0.0432 \times 0.000012 = 0.0000005184$

CARRYING IN MULTIPLICATION

In the process of multiplying, if two numbers multiplied together result in an answer that is larger than 9, part of the answer needs to be carried to the next place value. This is similar to carrying explained in Section 2: Addition of Decimals.

Example 11

This problem is completed in steps to show carrying in the multiplication process. Multiply 6.87 by 5.2.

```
   1
 6.87
× 5.2
    4
```

The numbers are positioned for multiplication without regard to their decimal points. Multiplication starts from the right by multiplying 2 times 7. The answer is 14. The 4 is placed under the 2, and the 1 is carried to the next column.

```
 1 1
 6.87
× 5.2
   74
```

Now multiply 2 times 8 to get 16. The 1 that was carried is added to 16 to give an answer of 17. The 7 is placed in the column next to the 4 in the answer, and the 1 is carried to the next column.

```
 1 1
 6.87
× 5.2
 1374
```

Next, multiply 2 times 6 to get 12. The 1 that was carried is added to the 12 to give an answer of 13. Because there are no more columns to multiply by 2, 13 is placed to the left of the 7.

```
   3
 6.87
× 5.2
 1374
   50
```

The numbers that were carried are dropped, and 7 is multiplied by 5 to get 35. Put a zero in the units place of the second answer line because the multiplying number (5) is in the tens place. The 5 is placed in the column underneath the 7, and the 3 is carried to the next column.

```
 4 3
 6.87
× 5.2
 1374
  350
```

Now multiply 5 times 8 to get an answer of 40. The 3 that was carried is added to 40 to give 43. The 3 is placed next to the 5 in the answer, and the 4 is carried to the next column.

```
 4 3
 6.87
× 5.2
 1374
34350
```

Next, multiply 5 times 6 to get an answer of 30. The 4 that was carried is added to 30 to give 34. The 4 is placed next to the 3 in the answer, and the 3 is carried to the next column. Because there are no more numbers in that column, the 3 is brought down next to the 4.

```
 6.87
× 5.2
  1
 1374
34350
   24
```

The numbers that were carried are dropped.
Now the numbers are added together starting from the rightmost column. The answer to the first column is 4, which is placed at the bottom of the rightmost column. The numbers in the next column (7 and 5) are added to get 12. As in addition, the 2 is placed in the answer and the 1 is carried to the next column.

```
   6.87
 × 5.2
     1
   1374
  34350
  35724
```

Then the next column is added (1 + 3 + 3) to get an answer of 7. The 7 is placed in the answer next to the 2. There is no carrying at this point.
The next column (1 + 4) is added to get 5. The 5 is placed next to the 7 in the answer. The answer to the final column is 3, which is placed next to 5 in the answer.

The final task is to position the decimal point. There are two decimal places in the first number and one decimal place in the second number for a total of three decimal places. Starting at the right of the last digit in the answer, move the decimal point three places to the left to position it between the 5 and the 7: 35.724.

Thus, $6.87 \times 5.2 = 35.724$

Remember the following tips for multiplying decimals:

- Do not line up the decimal points as is done in addition and subtraction.
- Multiply the two numbers without regard to the decimal points.
- Count the number of decimal places in each of the numbers that were multiplied.
- Starting from the far right in the answer, move the decimal to the left the same number of decimal places.
- If necessary, add zeros to position the decimal point properly.
- If there is no whole number, add a leading zero.

WORKING WITH ZEROS IN MULTIPLICATION

Working with zeros sometimes causes confusion in the multiplication process. The zeros are necessary in the numbers because they ensure that the digits are in their proper place. There is a big difference between $12, $102, and $1002.

Do not ignore the zeros. Multiply with the zeros even though zero times any number is zero. Remember that the use of the zero is necessary to put the digits in their proper place value.

Example 12

In this example, the top number has a zero. Notice how this affects the multiplication. Multiply 8.03 by 5.4.

1 8.03 × 5.4 2	Position the numbers for multiplication without regard to the decimal points. Multiply 4 times 3 to get 12. Place the 2 under the 4 and carry the 1.
1 8.03 × 5.4 12	Now multiply 4 times 0 to get 0. Add the 1 that was carried to get 1. Place the 1 to the left of the 2 in the first line of the answer.
8.03 × 5.4 3212	Next, multiply 4 times 8 to get 32. Place 32 to the left of the 1 in the first line of the answer. Because the next step is to multiply by the second digit, remove the 1 that was carried.
1 8.03 × 5.4 3212 50	Multiply 5 times 3 to get 15. To position the second row properly, place a zero under the first digit of the first line of the answer. Place the 5 in the second line of the answer under the multiplying digit of 5. Carry the 1.
1 8.03 × 5.4 3212 150	Multiply 5 times 0 to get 0. Add the 1 that was carried to get 1. Place the 1 to the left of the 5 in the second line of the answer.
1 8.03 × 5.4 3212 40150	Multiply 5 times 8 to get 40. Place 40 in the second line of the answer to the left of the 1. Remove the 1 that was carried because it is no longer needed.
8.03 × 5.4 3212 40150 43362	Add the numbers in the answer to get 43362. Count the number of decimal points in the numbers being multiplied. There are two in the first number and one in the second number for a total of three. Starting with the 2 in the answer, move the decimal point three places to the left to position it between the 3s: 43.362.

Thus, $8.03 \times 5.4 = 43.362$

Example 13

In this example, the bottom number has a zero. Notice how this affects the multiplication. Multiply 2.87 by 6.09.

$$\begin{array}{r} {\scriptstyle 6} \\ 2.87 \\ \times\ 6.09 \\ \hline 3 \end{array}$$

Position the numbers for multiplication without regard to the decimal points. Multiply 9 times 7 to get 63. Place the 3 under the 9 and carry the 6.

$$\begin{array}{r} {\scriptstyle 7\ 6} \\ 2.87 \\ \times\ 6.09 \\ \hline 2583 \end{array}$$

Now multiply 9 times 8 to get 72. Add the 6 to get 78. Place the 8 next to the 3 in the first line of the answer and carry the 7. Multiply 9 times 2 to get 18. Add the 7 to get 25. Place 25 to the left of 8 in the first line of the answer.

$$\begin{array}{r} 2.87 \\ \times\ 6.09 \\ \hline 2583 \\ 00 \end{array}$$

Remove the numbers that were carried. Put a zero in the units place of the second answer line because the multiplying number is in the tens place. Now multiply the top number by zero. 0 times 7 is 0. Place the zero from the multiplication next to the first zero.

$$\begin{array}{r} 2.87 \\ \times\ 6.09 \\ \hline 2583 \\ 0000 \end{array}$$

Now multiply 0 times 8 to get 0. Place this zero next to the other zeros on the second line of the answer. Multiply 0 times 2 to get another 0. Place this zero next to the rest of the zeros on the second line of the answer.

$$\begin{array}{r} {\scriptstyle 4} \\ 2.87 \\ \times\ 6.09 \\ \hline 2583 \\ 0000 \\ 200 \end{array}$$

Because the third multiplying digit is in the hundreds place, put a zero in the tens place and the units place of the third answer line. Multiply the third digit of 6 times the first digit of the top number to get 42. Put the 2 next to the 0 in the tens place of the third answer line and carry the 4.

$$\begin{array}{r} {\scriptstyle 5\ 4} \\ 2.87 \\ \times\ 6.09 \\ \hline 2583 \\ 0000 \\ 172200 \\ \hline 174783 \end{array}$$

Now multiply the 6 times the next digit of 8 in the top number to get 48. Add the 4 that was carried to get 52. Place the 2 next to the 2 in the third answer line and carry the 5. Multiply the 6 times the last digit of 2 in the top number to get 12. Add the 5 that was carried to get 17. Place the 17 in the third answer line. Add the three answer lines to get 174783.

To position the decimal point in the answer, count the number of decimal places in the top and bottom numbers. There are four places. Starting with the 3, move the decimal point four places to the left to position it between the first 7 from the left and the 4: 17.4783.

Thus, $2.87 \times 6.09 = 17.4783$

Example 14

In this example, both the top and the bottom numbers have zeros. Notice how this affects the multiplication. Multiply 8.0907 by 3.005.

$$\begin{array}{r} \scriptstyle 3 \\ 8.0907 \\ \times\ 3.005 \\ \hline 5 \end{array}$$

Position the two numbers without regard to the decimal points. Multiply the first digit of 5 in the bottom number times the first digit of 7 in the top number to get 35. Put 5 in the units place of the first answer line and carry the 3.

$$\begin{array}{r} \scriptstyle 3 \\ 8.0907 \\ \times\ 3.005 \\ \hline 35 \end{array}$$

Now multiply 5 times the first 0 from the right in the top number to get 0. Add the 3 that was carried to get 3 and place this number next to the 5 in the first answer line.

$$\begin{array}{r} \scriptstyle 4\ \ 3 \\ 8.0907 \\ \times\ 3.005 \\ \hline 535 \end{array}$$

Next, multiply 5 times the 9 in the top number to get 45. Place the 5 next to the 3 in the answer line and carry the 4.

$$\begin{array}{r} \scriptstyle 4\ \ 3 \\ 8.0907 \\ \times\ 3.005 \\ \hline 4535 \end{array}$$

Now multiply 5 times the second 0 in the top number to get 0. Add the 4 that was carried to get 4 and place this number next to the 5 on the first answer line.

$$\begin{array}{r} \scriptstyle 4\ \ 3 \\ 8.0907 \\ \times\ 3.005 \\ \hline 404535 \end{array}$$

Next, multiply 5 times the 8 in the top number to get 40. Place this number next to the 4 in the first answer line.

$$\begin{array}{r} 8.0907 \\ \times\ 3.005 \\ \hline 404535 \\ 0 \end{array}$$

Remove the numbers that were carried. Because the next multiplying number is in the tens place, put a zero in the units place of the second answer line.

$$\begin{array}{r} 8.0907 \\ \times\ 3.005 \\ \hline 404535 \\ 000000 \end{array}$$

Next, multiply the second digit in the multiplying number, which is a zero, times each of the digits of the top number. The answers are zero because zero times any number is zero. Place the zeros in the second answer line.

$$\begin{array}{r} 8.0907 \\ \underline{\times\ 3.005} \\ 404535 \\ 000000 \\ 0000000 \end{array}$$

Because the third multiplying number is in the hundreds place, put zeros in the tens and units places of the third answer line. Multiply zero times the top number and place the zeros on the third answer line.

$$\begin{array}{r} {\scriptstyle 2} \\ 8.0907 \\ \underline{\times\ 3.005} \\ 404535 \\ 000000 \\ 0000000 \\ 21000 \end{array}$$

Because the multiplying digit is in the thousands place, put zeros in the hundreds, tens, and units places in the fourth answer line. Multiply 3 times 7 in the top number to get 21. Place the 1 in the fourth answer line and carry the 2. Multiply 3 times 0 to get 0 and add the 2 that was carried. Place 2 in the fourth answer line.

$$\begin{array}{r} {\scriptstyle 2\ \ 2} \\ 8.0907 \\ \underline{\times\ 3.005} \\ 404535 \\ 000000 \\ 0000000 \\ \underline{242721000} \\ 243125535 \end{array}$$

Next, multiply 3 times 9 to get 27. Place the 7 in the fourth answer line and carry the 2. Multiply 3 times 0 to get 0 and add the 2 that was carried. Place this number in the fourth answer line. Finally, multiply 3 times 8 to get 24. Place the 24 in the fourth answer line. Add all four answer lines to get 243125535. Starting with the 5 in the answer, move the decimal point seven places to the left to position it between the 4 and the 3: 24.3125535.

Thus, $3.005 \times 8.0907 = 24.3125535$

EXERCISES IN MULTIPLYING DECIMALS

(Answers are on page 76.)
Multiply these decimal problems.

1.	2.	3.	4.
1.21 × 3	72.1 × 0.4	0.121 × 0.4	5.14 × 0.23

5.	6.	7.	8.
0.00042 × 0.03	7.94 × 0.56	5.08 × 4.2	9.75 × 6.08

9.	10.	11.	12.
7.0804 × 86.07	6.094 × 5.07	900.87 × 0.62	40.308 × 3.04

SOLVING MULTIPLICATION APPLICATIONS

Multiplication application problems generally provide information about one item and ask for information representing several items. For instance, if one shirt costs $5, how much would three shirts cost? To solve this problem, multiply the cost of one shirt ($5) by the number of shirts (3) to get the cost of three shirts ($15).

Steps for Solving an Application Problem

Step 1: Read the problem carefully. Pay close attention to the numbers in the problem.

Step 2: Read the question carefully. What exactly is it looking for? What label will be used in the answer?

Step 3: Eliminate any unnecessary information.

Step 4: Draw a diagram if it is helpful.

Step 5: Decide how to solve the problem. Some problems may require more than one step.

Step 6: Round the numbers to the highest place value and estimate the answer.

Step 7: Calculate the final answer and compare it with the estimate.

Step 8: Include the label in the answer.

Example 15

It takes 12 minutes to clean a patient's room. At this rate, how long will it take to clean four rooms?

Reason out the problem this way: If it takes 12 minutes to clean one room, it will take 2 times 12 minutes to clean two rooms, 3 times 12 minutes to clean three rooms, etc. The solution is to multiply the time it takes to clean one room times the number of rooms to be cleaned. In this problem, there are four rooms, so 4×12 min $= 48$ min.

Thus, at a rate of 12 minutes per room, it will take 48 minutes to clean four rooms.

Example 16

One pound is almost equal to 0.45 kg. If a person weighs 175 lb, how much does that person weigh in kilograms? (The symbol for "almost equal" is $\approx$.)

Reason out the problem this way: If 1 lb equals 0.45 kg, 2 lb will be 2 times 0.45 kg, 3 lb will be 3 times 0.45 kg, etc. The solution is to multiply the number of pounds times 0.45 kg. In this problem, there are 175 pounds, so 175 times 0.45 kg $\approx$ 78.75 kg.

Thus, if 1 lb is almost equal to 0.45 kg, 175 pounds will be almost equal to 78.75 kg.

Example 17

If a nurse was paid $31.50 an hour, how much did he earn in 7.5 hours?

Reason out the problem this way: If in one hour of work, the nurse was paid $31.50, for two hours of work, he is paid 2 times $31.50, for three hours of work he is paid 3 times $31.50, etc. The solution is to multiply the number of hours times the amount the nurse is paid an hour. So for 7.5 hours, multiply 7.5 times $31.50 to get $236.25.

Thus, working 7.5 hours for $31.50 an hour, the nurse earned $236.25.

Example 18

If one dosage of medication is 2.5 mL, how much medication is needed for 15 dosages?

Reason out the problem this way: If one dosage of medication is 2.5 mL, two dosages of medication is 2 times 2.5 mL, three dosages of medication is 3 times 2.5 mL, etc. The solution is to multiply the number of dosages times the amount of one dosage. Because this problem calls for 15 dosages, multiply 15 times 2.5. to get 37.5 mL.

Thus, 37.5 mL of medication is needed for 15 dosages.

EXERCISES IN MULTIPLICATION APPLICATIONS

(*Answers are on pages 76–78.*)

Solve these application problems using multiplication.

1. One dose of flu vaccine is 1.25 mL. How much vaccine is needed to vaccinate 30 walk-ins at a clinic?

2. How much does a package of 80 dosage spoons cost if each spoon costs $0.375?

3. A local food store can supply a nonprofit agency with individual fruit cups at a cost of $0.3125 if they are ordered in large numbers. How much will an order of 160 fruit cups cost?

4. How much of an experimental drug is needed if 1.5 mL injections are administered to 16 volunteers.

5. As a public service, a doctor's office charged $12.50 for a flu shot. How much money will the doctor collect for 312 shots?

6. To calculate the area of a rectangular room, multiply its length times its width. What is the area of a patient's hospital room that measures 3.81 meters by 3.048 meters? (The answer is in square meters.)

7. What is the area of a rectangular hospital closet that measures 2.75 meters by 1.6 meters? (The answer is in square meters.)

8. A nurse is paid $26.47 an hour. How much money will she make in 6.25 hours?

9. It takes 1.6 square yards of material to make one scrub top. If the material sells for $6.95 a square yard, how much will one scrub top cost?

10. Crafting materials from a craft supply store cost $3.48 a pound. How much will it cost a nursing home to buy 14.75 pounds of this crafting material?

11. If one day's supply of bandages costs $5.25, how much will a 14-day supply of bandages cost?

12. A case manager charges $84.75 an hour to oversee the care of an elderly resident in a long-term care facility. If the case manager worked with this resident 3.25 hours in one month, how much did she charge?

13. A case manager charges $84.75 an hour. How much would the case manager charge if she worked 12.75 hours on a case?

EXERCISES IN MIXED APPLICATIONS

(*Answers are on pages 78–80.*)

Solve these application problems using addition, subtraction, and/or multiplication.

1. One nurse is paid $21.86 an hour, and another nurse is paid $23.41 an hour. What is their difference in pay?

2. A tablet contains 2.3 mg of an antibiotic. A patient received two tablets twice a day for 14 days. How much antibiotic did the patient receive? (This is a multistep problem)

3. A patient paid a $55.00 doctor's bill for treatment of his back injury. The patient also bought a back brace for $18.99 and some ointment for $3.29. How much did the patient pay?

4. A patient was brought to the emergency room with a temperature of 102.1°F. After cold therapy, the patient's temperature was 99.7°F. By how much did the patient's temperature drop?

5. A doctor prescribed three 2.4 mL dosages of medication. If the container held 8 mL of medication, how much medication was left in the container? (This is a multistep problem.)

6. An attendant charged two male patients $12.50 each for haircuts. The attendant charged three female patients $24.50 each for hair coloring. What was the total bill? (This is a multistep problem.)

7. Physical therapy for a patient costs $65.75 an hour. If a patient receives 1.25 hours of therapy for 15 days, how much will the therapy cost? (Round to the nearest penny. This is a multistep problem.)

8. A nurse who makes $27.83 an hour worked 4.75 hours. The nurse's aide who works with the nurse makes $15.27 an hour and worked 6.5 hours. Compared to the nurse's aide, how much more did the nurse make? (Round to the nearest penny. This is a multistep problem.)

9. Scrub tops and bottoms are sold as a set for $17.99. Scrub tops are sold separately for $9.99, and scrub bottoms are sold separately for $8.99. If a medical assistant bought four sets of scrubs, how much would he save by buying them as a set instead of buying them separately? (This is a multistep problem.)

10. Who makes more—a doctor who works 2.75 hours for $86.00 an hour or a nurse who works 7.5 hours for $31.55 an hour? How much more does this person make? (Round to the nearest penny. This is a multistep problem.)

SECTION TEST: MULTIPLYING DECIMALS

(*Answers are on pages 80–81.*)

1. Multiply 12.4 by 3.1.

2. Multiply 6.89 by 7.5.

3. Multiply 0.987 by 0.23.

4. Multiply 0.028 by 0.028.

5. Multiply 0.0008 by 0.002.

6. Multiply 70 by 0.7.

7. Multiply 0.30906 by 0.79.

8. Multiply 0.9571 by 0.2008.

9. A tablet contains 0.5 mg of medication. See note page 47. A patient receives 1.5 tablets 3 times a day for four days. How many milligrams of medication did he receive?

10. A patient receives a dosage of 5.5 mL of medication 6 times every day. How much medication would the patient receive in seven days?

11. A case of saline solution is packaged in 0.5 liter bottles. If 24 bottles are in a case, how many liters of saline are in six cases?

12. 1 mL equals 0.001 liter. How many l iters are in 3.75 mL?

13. A nurse's normal pay is $32.80 an hour. She is paid 1.5 times her normal pay if she works overtime. How much will she be paid if she works one hour of overtime?

ANSWERS TO EXERCISES IN MULTIPLYING DECIMALS

(Exercises are on page 69.)

1. $$\begin{array}{r} 1.21 \\ \underline{\times 3} \\ 3.63 \end{array}$$

2. $$\begin{array}{r} 72.1 \\ \underline{\times 0.4} \\ 28.84 \end{array}$$

3. $$\begin{array}{r} 0.121 \\ \underline{\times 0.4} \\ 0.0484 \end{array}$$

4. $$\begin{array}{r} 5.14 \\ \underline{\times 0.23} \\ 1542 \\ \underline{10280} \\ 1.1822 \end{array}$$

5. $$\begin{array}{r} 0.00042 \\ \underline{\times 0.03} \\ 0.0000126 \end{array}$$

6. $$\begin{array}{r} 7.94 \\ \underline{\times 0.56} \\ 4764 \\ \underline{39700} \\ 4.4464 \end{array}$$

7. $$\begin{array}{r} 5.08 \\ \underline{\times 4.2} \\ 1016 \\ \underline{20320} \\ 21.336 \end{array}$$

8. $$\begin{array}{r} 9.75 \\ \underline{\times 6.08} \\ 7800 \\ 0000 \\ \underline{585000} \\ 59.2800 \end{array}$$

For problem 8, the last two zeros are dropped. The answer is 59.28.

9. $$\begin{array}{r} 7.0804 \\ \underline{\times 86.07} \\ 495628 \\ 000000 \\ 42482400 \\ \underline{566432000} \\ 609.410028 \end{array}$$

10. $$\begin{array}{r} 6.094 \\ \underline{\times 5.07} \\ 42658 \\ 00000 \\ \underline{3047000} \\ 30.89658 \end{array}$$

11. $$\begin{array}{r} 900.87 \\ \underline{\times 0.62} \\ 180174 \\ \underline{5405220} \\ 558.5394 \end{array}$$

12. $$\begin{array}{r} 40.308 \\ \underline{\times 3.04} \\ 161232 \\ 000000 \\ \underline{12092400} \\ 122.53632 \end{array}$$

ANSWERS TO EXERCISES IN MULTIPLICATION APPLICATIONS

(Exercises are on pages 71–72.)

1. $$\begin{array}{r} 1.25 \\ \underline{\times 30} \\ 000 \\ \underline{3750} \\ 37.50 \end{array}$$

If one dose of vaccine is 1.25 mL, 30 times this dose is needed for the walk-ins. 1.25 mL × 30 = 37.50 mL. In reporting the answer, the unnecessary zero is removed. 37.5 mL of vaccine is needed for the 30 walk-ins.

2. $$\begin{array}{r} 0.375 \\ \underline{\times 80} \\ 000 \\ \underline{30000} \\ 30.000 \end{array}$$

If 1 dosage spoon costs $0.375, multiply by 80 to find the cost of the package (80 spoons in a package). $0.375 times 80 equals $30. The extra zeros are dropped. The package of dosage spoons costs $30.

3. $$\begin{array}{r} 0.3125 \\ \underline{\times 160} \\ 0000 \\ 187500 \\ \underline{312500} \\ 50.0000 \end{array}$$

Multiply the cost of the fruit cups by the number of cups to find the cost of this order of fruit cups. $0.3125 × 160 = $50. The extra zeros are dropped. The order of 160 fruit cups will cost $50.

4.	1.5 × 16 90 150 24.0	Multiply 1.5 mL by 16 to find out how much of the drug is needed. 1.5 mL × 16 = 24 mL. The extra zero is dropped. 24 mL of the drug is needed.
5.	$12.50 × 312 2500 12500 375000 3900.00	If $12.50 is charged for one flu shot, the charges for 312 flu shots are 312 times as much. $12.50 × 312 = $3900.00. The doctor will collect $3900 for 312 flu shots.
6.	3.048 × 3.81 3048 243840 914400 11.61288	It does not matter which number is placed on top for multiplication. Generally, the number that has more digits is placed on top. 3.048 meters × 3.81 meters = 11.61288 square meters. When meters times meters is multiplied, the answer is square meters. The area of the patient's hospital room is 11.61288 square meters.
7.	2.75 × 1.6 1650 2750 4.400	Multiply length times width, as was done in problem 6, to find the area. 2.75 meters × 1.6 meters = 4.4 square meters. The unnecessary zeros are dropped. The area of the hospital closet is 4.4 square meters.
8.	$26.47 × 6.25 13235 52940 1588200 165.4375	Multiply the amount the nurse makes in one hour by the number of hours the nurse worked to find her pay. $26.47 × 6.25 = $165.4375. This number needs to be rounded to the nearest penny. $165.4375 rounds to $165.44, which is how much the nurse will make in 6.25 hours.
9.	$6.95 × 1.6 4170 6950 11.120	Multiply the amount of material by the cost per yard to find the total cost of one scrub. Drop the unnecessary zero. $6.95 × 1.6 = $11.12. One scrub will cost $11.12.
10.	14.75 × $3.48 11800 59000 442500 51.3300	Multiply the number of pounds of crafting material by the cost of 1 pound to find the total cost. 14.75 × $3.48 = $51.33. Drop the unnecessary zeros. It will cost $51.33 to buy 14.75 pounds of crafting material.

11. $$\begin{array}{r} \$5.25 \\ \underline{\times\ 14} \\ 2100 \\ \underline{5250} \\ \$73.50 \end{array}$$

Multiply the cost of one day's supply of bandages by 14 days to find the cost of the 14-day supply. The bandages will cost $73.50.

12. $$\begin{array}{r} \$84.75 \\ \underline{\times\ 3.25} \\ 42375 \\ 169500 \\ \underline{2542500} \\ 275.4375 \end{array}$$

Multiply the charge for one hour by the number of hours. $84.75 × 3.25 hours = $275.4375. Round this number to the nearest penny. $275.4375 rounds to $275.44, which is how much the case manager charged.

13. $$\begin{array}{r} \$84.75 \\ \underline{\times\ 12.75} \\ 42375 \\ 593250 \\ 169500 \\ \underline{8475000} \\ 1080.5625 \end{array}$$

Solve this problem the same way problem 12 was solved. The answer of $1080.5625 needs to be rounded to the nearest penny. The case manager would charge $1080.56.

ANSWERS TO EXERCISES IN MIXED APPLICATIONS

(Exercises are on pages 73–74.)

1. $$\begin{array}{r} \$23.41 \\ \underline{-\ \$21.86} \\ \$1.55 \end{array}$$

This is a subtraction problem. Subtract the smaller amount from the larger amount. The difference in pay is $1.55.

2. $$\begin{array}{r} 2.3 \\ \underline{\times\ 56} \\ 138 \\ \underline{+\ 1150} \\ 128.8 \end{array}$$

This is a multistep problem. The patient was given two tablets 2 times a day for 14 days. 2 × 2 × 14 = 56 tablets. Multiply 56 tablets times 2.3 mg of medication in each tablet to find the total amount of medication the patient received. The patient received 128.8 mg of medication.

3. $$\begin{array}{r} \$55.00 \\ \$18.99 \\ \underline{+\ \$3.29} \\ \$77.28 \end{array}$$

This is an addition problem. Add the doctor's bill, the cost of the back brace, and the cost of the ointment to find the total amount the patient paid. The patient paid $77.28.

4. $$\begin{array}{r} 102.1°\text{F} \\ \underline{-\ 99.7°\text{F}} \\ 2.4°\text{F} \end{array}$$

This is a subtraction problem. Subtract the current temperature from the original temperature to find how much the patient's temperature dropped. The patient's temperature dropped 2.4°F.

5. First, multiply the 2.4 mL of medication in one dosage times three dosages to find the total amount of medication given. Then subtract the amount of medication given from the total amount of medication in the container. There was 0.8 mL left in the container.

$$\begin{array}{r} 2.4 \text{ mL} \\ \times\ 3 \quad\ \ \\ \hline 7.2 \text{ mL} \end{array} \qquad \begin{array}{r} 8.0 \text{ mL} \\ -\ 7.2 \text{ mL} \\ \hline 0.8 \text{ mL} \end{array}$$

6. First, multiply 2 times \$12.50 to find the cost of the haircuts for the two male patients. Then multiply 3 times \$24.50 to find the cost of the hair coloring for the three female patients. Finally, add both answers to find the total cost. The total bill was \$98.50.

$$\begin{array}{r} \$12.50 \\ \times\ 2 \\ \hline \$25.00 \end{array} \qquad \begin{array}{r} \$24.50 \\ \times\ 3 \\ \hline \$73.50 \end{array} \qquad \begin{array}{r} \$25.00 \\ +\ \$73.50 \\ \hline \$98.50 \end{array}$$

7. First, multiply the cost per hour times the number of hours and round to the nearest penny. Then multiply this amount by the number of days to find the total cost of therapy for the patient. The total cost is \$1232.85.

cost for 1 day

$$\begin{array}{r} \$65.75 \\ \times\ 1.25 \\ \hline 32875 \\ 131500 \\ 657500 \\ \hline \$82.1875 \\ \textit{rounded: } \$82.19 \end{array}$$

cost for 15 days

$$\begin{array}{r} \$82.19 \\ \times\ 15 \\ \hline 41095 \\ 82190 \\ \hline \$1232.85 \end{array}$$

8. First, calculate the money the nurse made. Then calculate the money the nurse's aide made. Be sure to round to the nearest penny. Finally, subtract the nurse's aide's pay from the nurse's pay. The nurse earned \$32.93 more.

nurse's pay

$$\begin{array}{r} \$27.83 \\ \times\ 4.75 \\ \hline 13915 \\ 194810 \\ 1113200 \\ \hline 132.1925 \\ \textit{rounded: } \$132.19 \end{array}$$

nurse's aide's pay

$$\begin{array}{r} \$15.27 \\ \times\ 6.5 \\ \hline 7635 \\ 91620 \\ \hline 99.255 \\ \textit{rounded: } \$99.26 \end{array}$$

difference

$$\begin{array}{r} \$132.19 \\ -\ \$99.26 \\ \hline \$32.93 \end{array}$$

9. First, calculate how much four sets of scrubs cost. Then calculate how much four tops cost and how much four bottoms cost. Add the cost of the tops and bottoms to find how much the scrubs cost if bought separately. Finally, subtract the cost of the sets from the cost if bought separately. Buying the scrubs as a set would save the medical assistant $3.96.

cost of 4 sets	*cost of 4 tops*	*cost of 4 bottoms*	*cost of tops and bottoms*	*difference*
$17.99	$9.99	$8.99	$39.96	$75.92
× 4	× 4	× 4	+ $35.96	– $71.96
$71.96	$39.96	$35.96	$75.92	$3.96

10. First, calculate the doctor's pay and then the nurse's pay. Round to the nearest penny and drop any unnecessary zeros. Determine which pay is larger. Subtract the smaller pay from the larger pay to find the difference. The nurse makes $0.13 more than the doctor.

doctor's pay	*nurse's pay*	*difference*
$86.00	$31.55	$236.63
× 2.75	× 7.5	– $236.50
43000	15775	$0.13
602000	202850	
1720000	$236.625	
$236.5000	*rounded:* $236.63	
rounded: $236.50		

ANSWERS TO SECTION TEST: MULTIPLYING DECIMALS

(Section Test is on page 75.)

1.	2.	3.	4.
12.4	6.89	0.987	0.028
× 3.1	× 7.5	× 0.23	× 0.028
124	3445	2961	224
3720	48230	19740	560
38.44	51.675	0.22701	0.000784

5.	6.	7.	8.
0.0008	70	0.30906	0.9571
× 0.002	× 0.7	× 0.79	× 0.2008
0.0000016	49.0	278154	76568
		2163420	00000
		0.2441574	000000
			19142000
			0.19218568

Note: For problem 6, the answer is 49.

9. Multiply the 0.5 mg of medication times the 1.5 tablets to find the amount of milligrams in one dosage. Then multiply that answer by 3 to find the dosage for one day. Finally, multiply the answer by 4 to find the dosage for four days. Over this time period, the patient received 9 mg.

one dosage	*3 times a day*	*for 4 days*
$\begin{array}{r} 1.5 \\ \times\ 0.5 \\ \hline 0.75 \end{array}$	$\begin{array}{r} 0.75 \\ \times\ 3 \\ \hline 2.25 \end{array}$	$\begin{array}{r} 2.25 \\ \times\ 4 \\ \hline 9.00 \end{array}$

10. Multiply one dosage of 5.5 mL by 6 to find the amount of medication given in one day. Then multiply that answer by 7 to find the amount of medication given in seven days. The answer is 231 mL.

one dosage	*for 7 days*
$\begin{array}{r} 5.5 \\ \times\ 6 \\ \hline 33.0 \end{array}$	$\begin{array}{r} 33 \\ \times\ 7 \\ \hline 231 \end{array}$

11. Multiply the size of one bottle times the number of bottles in the case; then multiply by the number of cases. There are 72 liters of saline in the 6 cases.

one case	*all 6 cases*
$\begin{array}{r} 24 \\ \times\ 0.5 \\ \hline 12.0 \end{array}$	$\begin{array}{r} 12 \\ \times\ 6 \\ \hline 72 \end{array}$

12. $\begin{array}{r} 3.75 \\ \times\ 0.001 \\ \hline 0.00375 \end{array}$

1 mL = 0.001 L. Thus, multiply 0.001 times 3.75 to find the equivalent of 3.75 mL in liters. 3.75 mL = 0.00375 L

13. $\begin{array}{r} \$32.80 \\ \times\ 1.5 \\ \hline 1640 \\ 32800 \\ \hline \$49.200 \end{array}$

Because the nurse is paid $32.80 for one hour, the overtime is 1.5 times as much. Multiply $32.80 times 1.5 to find the overtime pay for one hour. The nurse will be paid $49.20 for one hour of overtime.

SECTION 5

Division of Decimals

OBJECTIVES

Upon completion of this section, you should be able to:

1. Explain the division process.
2. Remove a decimal point from the divisor and reposition the decimal point in the dividend.
3. Divide a number by a decimal number.
4. Work with zeros in the division process.
5. Work with remainders in the division process.
6. Divide a number to a fixed place accuracy.
7. Divide by a power of 10.
8. Solve application problems using division.

DIVISION CONCEPTS

Division of decimals is similar to division of whole numbers. The only real difference is the positioning of the decimal point in the answer. The number being divided is called the **dividend.** The number being divided into the dividend is called the **divisor.** The answer is the **quotient**. When a divisor does not divide evenly into the dividend, the leftover part is called a **remainder**.

Figure 5-1 shows the location of these terms in a division problem.

$$\text{Divisor}\overline{)\text{Dividend}}^{\text{Quotient}}$$

Figure 5-1

When dividing a decimal by a whole number, simply position the decimal point in the answer (quotient) directly above the decimal point in the number being divided (dividend).

Example 1

Divide 8.46 by 2.

```
   4.23
2)8.46
  8
  0 4
    4
    06
     6
     0
```

Figure 5-2

Step 1: Position the decimal point in the answer (quotient) so that it is above the decimal point in the dividend.

Step 2: Divide 2 into 8. It goes 4 times. Place the digit 4 above the 8 in the dividend (Figure 5-2).

Step 3: Multiply 4 times 2 (divisor) to get 8. Place the digit 8 under the 8 in the dividend. Subtract 8 from 8 to get 0.

Step 4: Bring the 4 down. Divide 2 into 4. It goes 2 times. Place the digit 2 above the 4 in the dividend.

Step 5: Multiply 2 times 2 to get 4. Place the digit 4 under the 4 in the dividend. Subtract 4 from 4 to get 0.

Step 6: Bring the 6 down. Divide 2 into 6. It goes 3 times. Place the digit 3 above the 6 in the dividend.

Step 7: Multiply 3 times 2 (divisor) to get 6. Place the digit 6 under the 6 in the dividend. Subtract 6 from 6 to get 0.

Thus: $8.46 \div 2 = 4.23$

Example 2

Divide 19.125 by 51. Figure 5-3A shows the beginning of the division problem, and Figure 5-3B shows the completed division problem.

Step 1: Position the decimal point in the quotient directly above the decimal point in the dividend.

Step 2: 51 does not divide into 1 or 19. Place a zero in the quotient directly above the 9 in the dividend.

Step 3: 51 does divide into 191. To estimate how many times 51 divides into 191, round 51 to 50. 50 divides into 191 at least 3 times but not 4 times; so 51 also should divide into 191 about 3 times. Place 3 in the quotient above the last 1 in 191.

Step 4: Multiply 3 times 51 to get 153. Write 153 under 191. (The spacing in the example may look a little strange. It has been adjusted so that the digits line up.)

Step 5: Subtract 153 from 191 to get 38 (Figure 5-3A).

Step 6: Bring down the 2. The working number is now 382.

```
     0.3
51)19.125
    15 3
     3 8
```

Figure 5-3A

Step 7: Use the same method in Step 1 to estimate how many times 51 divides into 382. It goes at least 7 times but not 8 times. Place 7 in the quotient above the 2 in the dividend.

Step 8: Multiply 7 times 51 to get 357. Write 357 under 382.

Step 9: Subtract 357 from 382 to get 25.

Step 10: Bring down the 5. The working number is now 255.

Step 11: Estimate how many times 51 divides into 255. It goes 5 times but not 6 times. Place 5 in the quotient above the 5 in the dividend.

Step 12: Multiply 5 times 51 to get 255. Write 255 under 255.

Step 13: Subtract to get 0 (Figure 5-3B).

Thus: $19.125 \div 51 = 0.375$

```
     0.375
51)19.125
    15 3
     3 82
     3 57
       255
       255
         0
```

Figure 5-3B

In this problem, it was correctly estimated that 51 would divide into 191 at least 3 times. If the estimation had been 2 instead of 3, the subtraction would have given an answer that was larger than the divisor (Figure 5-3C). If this occurs, the estimation is too small. Try a larger number.

```
     0.2
51)19.125
    10 2
     8 9
```

Figure 5-3C

If the estimation had been 4 instead of 3, the multiplied number would have been larger than 191 and subtraction would not have been possible (Figure 5-3D). If this occurs, the estimation is too large. Try a smaller number.

```
     0.4
51)19.125
    20 4
```

Figure 5-3D

EXERCISES IN DIVIDING DECIMALS BY WHOLE NUMBERS

(*Answers are on page 110.*)

Divide these decimal numbers by the whole numbers. The answers will not have remainders. Remember to drop extra zeros in the answer.

1. $87.4 \div 2$
2. $9.639 \div 3$
3. $8.48 \div 4$
4. $47.6 \div 7$
5. $60.8 \div 8$
6. $98.61 \div 19$
7. $94.6 \div 22$
8. $156.8 \div 49$
9. $82.8 \div 36$

POSITIONING THE DECIMAL POINT IN DIVISION

> When a number is divided by a decimal, the decimal must be removed from the divisor. First, move the decimal point to the position just after the last digit in the divisor. Then discard any leading zeros in the divisor. Finally, move the decimal in the dividend the same number of places to the right as was done with the divisor. Add zeros to create decimal places if necessary. Place the decimal point in the quotient (answer) directly above the decimal point in the dividend. It is important to move the decimal point the same number of places in both the divisor and the dividend.

Example 3

Remove the decimal point from the divisor and reposition the decimal point in the dividend in this problem: 9.312 ÷ 1.6. Do not complete the division.

Step 1: Position the numbers in the division problem (Figure 5-4A).

$1.6\overline{)9.312}$

Figure 5-4A

Step 2: Move the decimal point in the divisor (1.6) one place to the right so that it is positioned just after the 6. When a decimal point is to the right of the last digit in a number, the decimal point usually is not shown.

Step 3: Move the decimal point in the dividend (9.312) one place to the right so that it is positioned between the 3 and the 1 (Figure 5-4B).

$16.\overline{)93.12}$

Figure 5-4B

Example 4

Remove the decimal point from the divisor and reposition the decimal point in the dividend in this problem: 29.495 ÷ 0.85. Do not complete the division.

Step 1: Position the numbers in the division problem (Figure 5-5A).

$0.85\overline{)29.495}$

Figure 5-5A

Step 2: Move the decimal point in the divisor (0.85) two places to the right so that it is positioned just after the 5.

Step 3: Remove the leading zero from 085.

Step 4: Move the decimal point in the dividend (29.495) two places to the right so that it is positioned between the 9 and the 5 (Figure 5-5B).

$85.\overline{)2949.5}$

Figure 5-5B

Note: Move the decimal point in the dividend the same number of places to the right as was done in the divisor. Moving the decimal point this way does not change the final answer.

Example 5

Remove the decimal point from the divisor and reposition the decimal point in the dividend in this problem: 9 ÷ 0.0045. Do not complete the division.

Step 1: Position the numbers in the division problem (Figure 5-6A).

$0.0045\overline{)9}$

Figure 5-6A

Step 2: Move the decimal point in the divisor (0.0045) four places to the right so that it is positioned just after the 5.

Step 3: Remove the three leading zeros from 00045.

Step 4: Move the decimal point in the dividend (9) four places to the right. Add the necessary four zeros to the right of the 9 (Figure 5-6B).

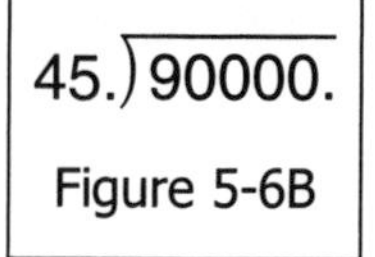

Figure 5-6B

Example 6

Divide 1.575 by 0.21. Remove the decimal point from the divisor, reposition the decimal point in the dividend, and divide to get the answer.

Step 1: Position the numbers in the division problem (Figure 5-7A).

$0.21\overline{)1.575}$

Figure 5-7A

Step 2: Move the decimal point in the divisor (0.21) two places to the right so that it is positioned just after the 1.

Step 3: Remove the leading zero from 021.

Step 4: Move the decimal point in the dividend (1.575) two places to the right so that it is positioned just after the 7. The number is 157.5 (Figure 5-7B).

Step 5: Position the decimal point in the quotient (answer) just above the decimal point in the dividend (Figure 5-7B).

$21.\overline{)157.5}$

Figure 5-7B

(Figure 5-7C shows the completed problem.)

Step 6: Because 21 does not divide into 15, divide 21 into 157. Estimate the answer of 20 into 150 as 7.

Step 7: Place 7 above the 7 in the dividend. Multiply 7 times 21 and place the answer of 147 underneath 157 in the dividend.

Step 8: Subtract 147 from 157 to get 10. Bring down the 5.

Step 9: Divide 21 into 105. Estimate the answer of 20 into 105 as 5.

Step 10: Place 5 above the 5 in the dividend. Multiply 5 times 21 and place the answer of 105 underneath 105.

$$\begin{array}{r} 7.5 \\ 21.\overline{)157.5} \\ \underline{147} \\ 10\ 5 \\ \underline{10\ 5} \\ 0 \end{array}$$

Figure 5-7C

Step 11: Subtract 105 from 105 to get 0.

Thus: 1.575 divided by 0.21 is 7.5

Example 7

Divide 3.087 by 0.049.

Step 1: Position the numbers in the division problem (Figure 5-8A).

$$0.049\overline{)3.087}$$

Figure 5-8A

Step 2: Move the decimal point in the divisor (0.049) three places to the right so that it is positioned just after the 9.

Step 3: Remove the two leading zeros from 0049.

Step 4: Move the decimal point in the dividend (3.087) three places to the right so that it is positioned just after the 7. The number is 3087.

Step 5: Position the decimal point in the quotient (answer) just above the decimal point in the dividend. (Figure 5-8B).

$$\begin{array}{r} . \\ 49.\overline{)3087.} \end{array}$$

Figure 5-8B

(Figure 5-7C shows the completed problem.)

Step 6: Because 49 does not divide into 30, divide 49 into 308. Estimate the answer of 50 into 308 as 6.

Step 7: Place 6 above the 8 in the dividend. Multiply 6 times 49 and place the answer of 294 underneath 308 in the dividend.

Step 8: Subtract 294 from 308 to get 14. Bring down the 7.

Step 9: Divide 49 into 147. Estimate the answer of 50 into 147 as 3.

Step 10: Place 3 above the 7 in the dividend. Multiply 3 times 49 and place the answer of 147 underneath 147.

$$\begin{array}{r} 63. \\ 49.\overline{)3087.} \\ \underline{294} \\ 147 \\ \underline{147} \\ 0 \end{array}$$

Figure 5-8C

Step 11: Subtract 147 from 147 to get 0.

Thus: 3.087 divided by 0.049 is 63

EXERCISES IN DIVIDING A NUMBER BY A DECIMAL

(Answers are on page 110.)

Divide these numbers by the decimals.

1. $33 \div 2.2$
2. $4 \div 0.25$
3. $49.8 \div 0.6$
4. $0.18 \div 0.12$
5. $4.52 \div 0.4$
6. $5.12 \div 0.8$
7. $0.041 \div 0.05$
8. $0.0096 \div 0.003$
9. $0.224 \div 0.016$

QUOTIENTS WITH ZEROS IN THE MIDDLE

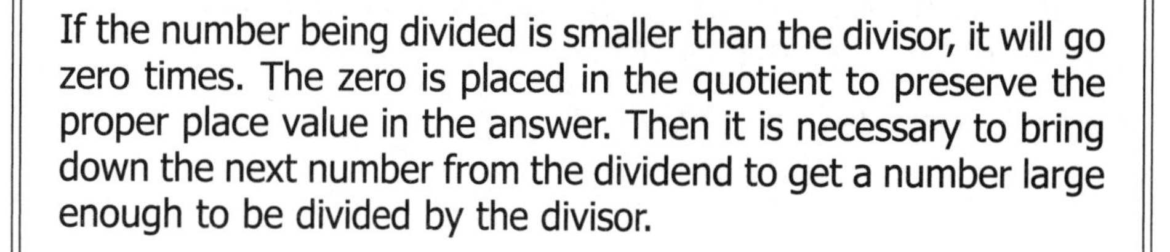
If the number being divided is smaller than the divisor, it will go zero times. The zero is placed in the quotient to preserve the proper place value in the answer. Then it is necessary to bring down the next number from the dividend to get a number large enough to be divided by the divisor.

Example 8

Figure 5-9A shows a partially completed division problem.

The next step in the problem is to divide 12 into 6. Because 12 does not divide into 6, place a 0 above the 6 in the dividend. Bring down the 0 in the dividend. Then divide 12 into 60. (Figure 5-9B shows the completed problem.)

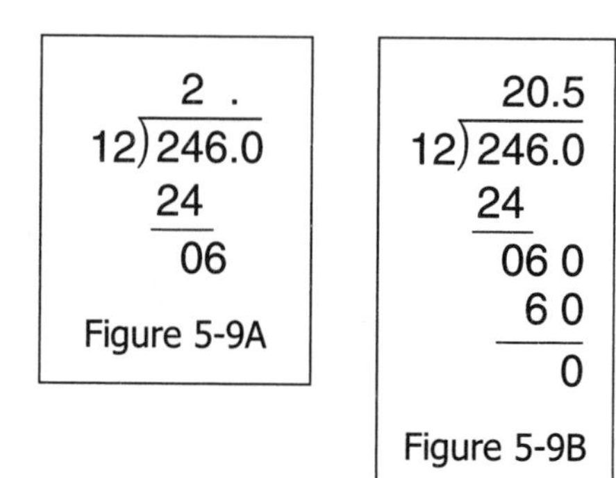

Figure 5-9A

Figure 5-9B

Example 9

Divide 17.661 by 8.7. Notice how a zero is used in the quotient.

Step 1: Position the numbers in the division problem (Figure 5-10A).

Step 2: Move the decimal point in the divisor (8.7) one place to the right to position it to the right of 7.

Step 3: Move the decimal point one place to the right in the dividend so that it is between the 6s.

Step 4: Position the decimal point in the quotient (answer) just above the decimal point in the dividend (Figure 5-10B).

(Figure 5-10C shows the completed problem.)

Step 5: Because 87 does not divide into 17, divide 87 into 176. It goes 2 times.

Step 6: Place 2 above the first 6 in the dividend. Multiply 2 times 87 and place the answer of 174 underneath 176 in the dividend.

Step 7: Subtract 174 from 176 to get 2. Bring down the 6.

Step 8: Because 87 does not divide into 26, place a 0 in the quotient above the second 6 in the dividend.

Step 9: Multiply 0 times 87 and place the answer of 0 underneath 26.

Step 10: Subtract 0 from 26 to get 26. Bring down the 1. Divide 87 into 261. It goes 3 times.

Step 11: Place 3 above the 1 in the dividend. Multiply 3 times 87 and place the answer of 261 underneath 261.

Step 12: Subtract 261 from 261 to get 0.

Thus: 17.661 divided by 8.7 is 2.03. If the zero had not been in the tenths place, the number would have been 2.3. 2.03 and 2.3 are completely different numbers.

```
8.7)17.661
```

Figure 5-10A

```
        .
87.)176.61
```

Figure 5-10B

```
      2.03
87.)176.61
    174
      2 6
        0
      261
      261
        0
```

Figure 5-10C

QUOTIENTS WITH ZEROS AT THE END

> A common error in division involves zeros at the end of the quotient. In some division problems, all nonzero digits in the dividend may be divided, yet zeros remain in the dividend. To maintain proper place value, it is necessary to complete the division process to get zeros in the quotient. The mistake some students make is stopping the division process too soon.

Example 10

Divide 1 by 0.0025. Notice how zeros are handled.

Step 1: Position the numbers in the division problem (Figure 5-11A).

$$0.0025\overline{)1}$$

Figure 5-11A

Step 2: Move the decimal point in the divisor (0.0025) four places to the right so that it is positioned just to the right of the 5.

Step 3: Remove the three leading zeros from 00025.

Step 4: The decimal point in the dividend (1) is just to the right of the 1. Move the decimal point four places to the right. To do this, add the necessary four zeros to the right of the 1 to ensure the proper place value. The number now becomes 10000.

Step 5: Position the decimal point in the quotient (answer) just above the decimal point in the dividend (Figure 5-11B).

(Figure 5-11C shows the completed problem.)

$$\begin{array}{r} . \\ 25.\overline{)10000.} \end{array}$$

Figure 5-11B

Step 6: Because 25 does not divide into 10, divide 25 into 100. It goes 4 times.

Step 7: Place 4 above the second zero in the dividend. Multiply 4 times 25 and place the answer of 100 underneath 100 in the dividend.

Step 8: Subtract 100 from 100 to get 0. A common mistake is thinking that the answer is complete. It isn't. There are still two zeros in the dividend. It is necessary to continue the division so that the answer has the proper place value.

Step 9: Bring down the next zero. Divide 25 into 00. It goes 0 times.

Step 10: Place 0 above the third 0 in the dividend. Multiply 0 times 25 and place the answer of 0 underneath 00.

$$\begin{array}{r} 400. \\ 25.\overline{)10000.} \\ \underline{100} \\ 00 \\ \underline{0} \\ 00 \\ \underline{0} \\ 0 \end{array}$$

Figure 5-11C

Step 11: Subtract 0 from 00 to get 0. Bring down the last zero. Divide 25 into 00. It goes 0 times.

Step 12: Place 0 above the last 0 in the dividend. Multiply 0 times 25 and place the answer of 0 underneath 00.

Step 13: Subtract 0 from 00 to get 0.

Thus: 1 divided by 0.0025 is 400

EXERCISES IN DIVIDING WITH ZEROS IN THE QUOTIENT

(*Answers are on page 110.*)

Divide these numbers by the decimals. The problems will have at least one zero in the quotient, but there are no remainders.

1. $8.12 \div 4$
2. $564.9 \div 7$
3. $6.1218 \div 6$
4. $117.117 \div 13$
5. $4.2112 \div 1.4$
6. $11.4113 \div 1.9$

WORKING WITH REMAINDERS

A **remainder** occurs when the divisor does not divide evenly into the dividend. Following are three methods of dealing with remainders:

- Show the remainder as a fraction, with the remainder as the numerator and the divisor as the denominator. Reduce the fraction if possible. To avoid having a decimal and a fraction in the same number, stop dividing before a decimal is in the quotient.
- Add zeros to the dividend and continue the division until there is no remainder.
- Round to a specific place value. This method is applicable to the healthcare professional who frequently rounds to the nearest tenth or hundredth.

Example 11

Divide 52.3 by 0.5. Show the remainder as a fraction with the answer.

Step 1: Position the numbers in the division problem (Figure 5-12A).

$0.5\overline{)52.3}$

Figure 5-12A

Step 2: Move the decimal point in the divisor (0.5) one place to the right so that it is positioned just after the 5.

Step 3: Remove the leading zero from 05.

Step 4: Move the decimal point in the dividend (52.3) one place to the right so that it is positioned just after the 3.

Step 5: Position the decimal point in the quotient (answer) just above the decimal point in the dividend (Figure 5-12B).

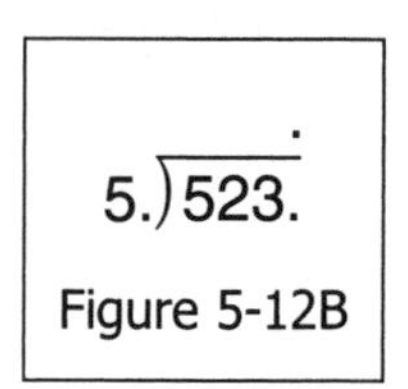
Figure 5-12B

(Figure 5-12C shows the completed problem.)

Step 6: Divide 5 into 5. It goes 1 time.

Step 7: Place 1 above the 5 in the dividend. Multiply 1 times 5 and place the answer of 5 underneath the 5 in the dividend.

```
   104.
5.)523.
   5
   02
    0
    23
    20
     3
```

Figure 5-12C

Step 8: Subtract 5 from 5 to get 0. Bring down the 2.

Step 9: Because 5 does not divide into 2, place 0 above the 2 in the dividend.

Step 10: Multiply 0 times 5 and place the answer of 0 underneath 02. Subtract 0 from 02 to get 2. Bring down the 3.

Step 11: Divide 5 into 23. It goes 4 times. Place the 4 above the 3 in the dividend.

Step 12: Multiply 4 times 5 and put the answer of 20 under 23. Subtract 20 from 23 and put the answer of 3 under 20.

Step 13: The remainder is 3. To show this as a fraction, put the remainder (3) in the numerator and the divisor (5) in the denominator to get the fraction $\frac{3}{5}$ Eliminate the decimal between 104 and the fraction $\frac{3}{5}$ in the final answer.

Thus: 5.23 divided by 0.5 is $104\frac{3}{5}$ This remainder is shown as a fraction. Reduce the fraction if possible. Avoid a fraction with a decimal.

Example 12

Divide 0.33 by 8.8. Show the remainder as a decimal in the answer.

Step 1: Position the numbers in the division problem. (Figure 5-13A).

$$8.8\overline{)0.33}$$

Figure 5-13A

Step 2: Move the decimal point in the divisor (8.8) one place to the right so that it is positioned just after the last 8.

Step 3: Move the decimal point in the dividend (0.33) one place to the right so that it is positioned just after the first 3.

Step 4: Position the decimal point in the quotient (answer) just above the decimal point in the dividend. (Figure 5-13B).

$$\begin{array}{r} . \\ 88.\overline{)3.3} \end{array}$$

Figure 5-13B

(Figure 5-13C shows the completed problem.)

Step 5: Because 88 will not divide into 33, add a 0 after the decimal point. (Zeros can be added after the decimal point without changing the number.) Divide 88 into 330. It goes 3 times.

Step 6: Place 3 above the first 0 in the dividend. Multiply 3 times 88 and place the answer of 264 underneath 330 in the dividend.

Step 7: Subtract 264 from 330 to get 66. Add another 0 to the dividend. Bring down the 0.

Step 8: Divide 88 into 660. It goes 7 times.

Step 9: Place 7 above the second 0 in the dividend. Multiply 7 times 88 and place the answer of 616 underneath 660.

$$\begin{array}{r} 0.0375 \\ 88.\overline{)3.3000} \\ \underline{2\ 64} \\ 660 \\ \underline{616} \\ 440 \\ \underline{440} \\ 0 \end{array}$$

Figure 5-13C

Step 10: Subtract 616 from 660 to get 44. Because there are no more digits in the dividend, add another zero.

Step 11: Divide 88 into 440. It goes 5 times. Place 5 above the last zero in the dividend.

Step 12: Multiply 5 times 88 and place the answer of 440 underneath 440.

Step 13: Subtract 440 from 440 to get a remainder of 0.

Thus: 0.33 divided by 8.8 is 0.0375. This answer does not have a remainder because zeros were added to the number being divided to get the final answer.

EXERCISES IN DIVIDING WITH REMAINDERS

(*Answers are on page 110.*)

Divide these numbers. Show remainders as fractions.

1. $16 \div 5$
2. $56 \div 17$
3. $7 \div 6$
4. $19 \div 4$
5. $9 \div 1.1$
6. $61 \div 21$

Divide these numbers. Add zeros to the dividend to get rid of the remainders.

7. $3 \div 4$
8. $3 \div 8$
9. $7 \div 8$
10. $3 \div 16$
11. $9 \div 16$
12. $11 \div 32$

Example 13

Sometimes adding zeros does not allow a division problem to yield an answer. Sometimes the division continues forever. Consider this example: divide 5 by 9.

Step 1: Position the numbers in the division problem.

Step 2: Because there is no decimal point in the divisor, no decimal points need to be moved. Place the decimal point in the answer (Figure 5-14A).

(Figure 5-14B shows the completed problem.)

$$9\overline{)5.}$$

Figure 5-14A

Step 3: Because 9 does not divide into 5, add a 0 after the decimal point. (Zeros can be added after the decimal point without changing the number.)

Step 4: Divide 9 into 50. It goes 5 times.

Step 5: Place 5 above the first 0 in the dividend. Multiply 5 times 9 and place the answer of 45 underneath 50 in the dividend.

Step 6: Subtract 45 from 50 to get 5. If the division were to continue with more zeros added to the dividend, 9 would always go into 50 five times, 5 times 9 would give 45, and 50 minus 45 would be 5.

```
   0.55
9)5.00
  4 5
   50
   45
    5
```

Figure 5-14B

Note: This answer is a repeating decimal. Repeating decimals may be shown with a bar above the digits that repeat ($0.\overline{5}$). Another method is to show the remainder as a fraction. In this case, 5 divided by 9 is $\frac{5}{9}$.

DIVIDING TO A FIXED PLACE ACCURACY

Health care professionals often work with medications that are rounded to the nearest tenth or hundredth. For example, a medication is administered at a rate of 1.8 mg per kg of body weight. A nurse calculates the dosage to be 0.0246575 mg; however, the medication can be administered only in hundredth increments. The answer must be rounded to the nearest hundredth. In this example, the nurse must divide to the nearest hundredth. Dividing to a specific place value is called **dividing to a fixed place accuracy**.

To divide to a fixed place accuracy, follow these steps:

Step 1: Determine how many places will be needed after the decimal point in the answer.

Step 2: Add one more place value for rounding purposes.

Step 3: Do the division. Ignore any remainder.

Step 4: Locate the digit in the specific place value to be rounded. This is the rounding digit.

Step 5A: Look at the digit directly to its right. If this digit is 5 or larger, increase the rounding digit by one.

Step 5B: If this digit is not 5 or larger, do not change the rounding digit. Drop all digits to the right of the rounding digit.

Example 14

Round 3.76 to the nearest tenth.

Step 1: Locate the digit in the tenths place. In 3.76, that digit is 7.

Step 2: Locate the digit to the right. If the digit is 5 or larger, add 1 to the 7. If the digit is not 5 or larger, drop all digits to the right of the 7. In this case, the digit 6 is 5 or larger; so 1 is added to 7.

Thus: 3.76 rounded to the nearest tenth is 3.8

Example 15

Round 4.32 to the nearest tenth.

Step 1: Locate the digit in the tenth's place. In 4.32, that digit is 3.

Step 2: Locate the digit to the right. If the digit is 5 or larger, add 1 to the 3. If the digit is not 5 or larger, drop all digits to the right of the 3. In this case, the digit 2 is not 5 or larger; so all digits to the right of 3 are dropped.

Thus: 4.32 rounded to the nearest tenth is 4.3

Example 16

Round 9.8476 to the nearest hundredth.

Step 1: Locate the digit in the hundredths place. In 9.8476, that digit is 4.

Step 2: Locate the digit to the right. If the digit is 5 or larger, add 1 to the 4. If the digit is not 5 or larger, drop all digits to the right of the 4. In this case, the digit 7 is 5 or larger; so 1 is added to 4.

Thus: 9.8476 rounded to the nearest hundredth is 9.85

Example 17

Round 5.6348 to the nearest hundredth.

Step 1: Locate the digit in the hundredths place. In 5.6348, that digit is 3.

Step 2: Locate the digit to the right. If the digit is 5 or larger, add 1 to the 3. If the digit is not 5 or larger, drop all digits to the right of the 3. In this case, the digit 4 is less than 5; so all digits to the right of 3 are dropped.

Thus: 5.6348 rounded to the nearest hundredth is 5.63

Example 18

Round 0.9998 to the nearest thousandth.

Step 1: Locate the digit in the thousandth's place. In 0.9998, that digit is the last 9.

Step 2: Locate the digit to the right. If the digit is 5 or larger, add 1 to the 9. If the digit is not 5 or larger, drop all digits to the right of the 9. In this case, the digit 8 is greater than 5; so 1 is added to the 9.

When 1 is added to the 9, the answer becomes 10. Because of place value, the 0 remains in the thousandth's place, 1 is added to the hundredth's place, and the process continues. In this case, when 1 is added to the thousandth's place, $0.999 + 0.001$ becomes 1.000. The zeros following the decimal point are dropped.

Thus: 0.9998 rounded to the nearest thousandth is 1.

Example 19

Divide 0.76 by 0.31 and round to the nearest tenth.

Step 1: Position the numbers for division.

Step 2: Move the decimal point in the divisor so that division is by a whole number. Place the decimal point in the answer (Figure 5-15A).

$31\overline{)76.}$

Figure 5-15A

Step 3: Determine how many places will be needed. In this case, one place is needed for the tenth's position, in addition to one more place for rounding. Add two zeros to the dividend (Figure 5-15B).

$31\overline{)76.00}$

Figure 5-15B

(Figure 5-15C shows the completed division.)

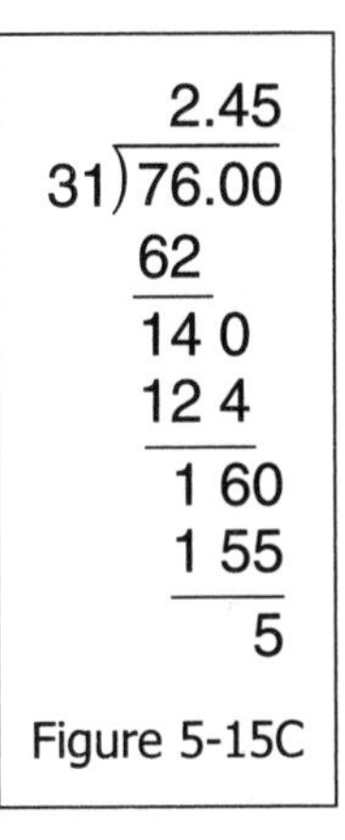

Figure 5-15C

Step 4: Do the division. 76.00 divided by 31 equals 2.45 with a remainder of 5.

Step 5: For rounding purposes, ignore the remainder. The instructions call for rounding the answer to the nearest tenth. The digit 4 is in the tenth's place. The digit to the right is 5, which is 5 or larger; so add 1 to the digit in the tenth's place.

Thus: 0.76 divided by 0.31, rounded to the nearest tenth, is 2.5

Example 20

Divide 0.76 by 0.31 and round to the nearest hundredth.

Step 1: Position the numbers for division.

Step 2: Move the decimal point in the divisor so that division is by a whole number. Place the decimal point in the answer (Figure 5-16A).

$31\overline{)76.}$

Figure 5-16A

Step 3: Determine how many places will be needed. In this case, two places are needed for the hundredth's position, in addition to one more place for rounding. Add three zeros to the dividend (Figure 5-16B).

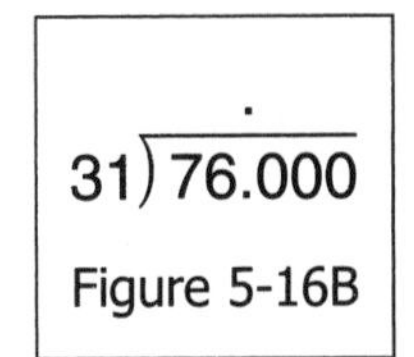

Figure 5-16B

(Figure 5-16C shows the completed division.)

```
      2.451
31)76.000
   62
   14 0
   12 4
    1 60
    1 55
       50
       31
       19
```

Figure 5-16C

Step 4: Do the division. 76.000 divided by 31 equals 2.451 with a remainder of 19.

Step 5: For rounding purposes, ignore the remainder. The instructions call for rounding the answer to the nearest hundredth. The digit 5 is in the hundredth's place. The digit to the right is 1, which is not 5 or larger; so the digits to the right of the hundredth's place are dropped.

Thus: 0.76 divided by 0.31, rounded to the nearest hundredth, is 2.45

EXERCISES IN DIVIDING TO A FIXED PLACE ACCURACY

(Answers are on pages 110–111.)

Round these answers to the nearest tenth.

1. $8 \div 7$
2. $8 \div 9$
3. $8 \div 3$

Round these answers to the nearest hundredth.

4. $5 \div 9$
5. $5 \div 7$
6. $5 \div 11$

Round these answers to the nearest thousandth.

7. $7 \div 11$
8. $7 \div 9$
9. $7 \div 13$

DIVIDING BY A POWER OF 10

A power of 10 is any number whose first digit is 1 and the remaining digits are zeros. These numbers are powers of 10: 10, 100, 1000, 10,000, etc.

To divide by a power of 10, count the number of zeros in the power of 10. Then move the decimal point to the left the same number of places. When a number is divided by a power of 10, the answer is smaller than the dividend. Moving the decimal point to the left results in a smaller answer. It may be necessary to add leading zeros.

Thus, to divide 12.34 by 10, move the decimal point one place to the left so that the number becomes 1.234. To divide that same number by 100, move the decimal point two places to the left so that the number becomes 0.1234. To divide the same number by 1000, move the decimal point three places to the left so that the number becomes 0.01234

Example 21

Divide 563.8 by 100.

Step 1: Determine whether the divisor is a power of 10. Because 100 has a 1 followed by zeros, it is a power of 10.

Step 2: Count the number of zeros in the power of 10. There are two zeros.

Step 3: Move the decimal point in the dividend two places to the left.

Thus: 563.8 divided by 100 is 5.638

Example 22

Divide 27.4 by 10,000.

Step 1: Determine whether the divisor is a power of 10. Because 10,000 has a 1 and is followed by zeros, it is a power of 10.

Step 2: Count the number of zeros in the power of 10. There are four zeros.

Step 3: Move the decimal point in the dividend four places to the left. Three leading zeros need to be added to the number.

Thus: 27.4 divided by 10,000 is 0.00274

EXERCISES IN DIVIDING BY A POWER OF 10

(*Answers are on page 111.*)

Divide these numbers by the power of 10 indicated.

1. $68.3 \div 10$
2. $8 \div 10$
3. $0.4 \div 10$
4. $128 \div 100$
5. $12.8 \div 100$
6. $0.17 \div 100$
7. $957.2 \div 1000$
8. $1.6 \div 1000$
9. $5 \div 1000$

SOLVING DIVISION APPLICATIONS

Division takes a larger quantity and divides it into an equal number of smaller parts. For example, if $20 is being evenly divided among five children, $20 would be divided by 5 to get an answer of $4. Thus, each child would get $4. To verify that this is correct, if the $4 from each child were combined together, there would be $20 ($\$4 \times 5 = \$20$).

Steps for Solving an Application Problem

Step 1: Read the problem carefully. Pay close attention to the numbers in the problem.

Step 2: Read the question carefully. What exactly is it looking for? What label will be used in the answer?

Step 3: Eliminate any unnecessary information.

Step 4: Draw a diagram if it is helpful.

Step 5: Decide how to solve the problem. Some problems may require more than one step.

Step 6: Round the numbers to the highest place value and estimate the answer.

Step 7: Calculate the final answer and compare it with the estimate.

Step 8: Include the label in the answer.

Example 23

1. *How many 1.2 oz doses of medication are in a 24 oz bottle of medication?*

One way to solve this problem is to physically pour 1.2 oz doses from the 24 oz bottle and count the number of doses. An easier way is to consider that the 24 oz of medication needs to be divided into 1.2 oz doses. 24 oz divided by 1.2 oz = 20 doses. (Figure 5-17 shows the completed problem.)

$$\begin{array}{r} 20. \\ 12\overline{)240.} \\ \underline{24} \\ 00 \\ \underline{0} \\ 0 \end{array}$$

Figure 5-17

EXERCISES IN DIVISION APPLICATIONS

(*Answers are on pages 111–112.*)

Solve these decimal applications.

1. If a doctor can examine a patient in 0.25 hours, how many patients can the doctor examine in 4.5 hours?
2. If a different doctor gives a more thorough exam to a patient in 0.75 hours, how many patients can this doctor examine in the same 4.5 hours?
3. A bottle holds 120 mL of medication. How many 1.5 mL doses are in the bottle?
4. A container holds 67.5 mL of a powerful disinfectant. If 4 mL are used for every liter of water in preparing a batch of cleaning solution, about how many complete batches of cleaning solution can be made from this container of disinfectant?
5. Nurses must monitor a patient around the clock. If five nurses are on duty for a 24-hour period, how many hours will each nurse monitor the patient if their time is split evenly?
6. A patient received 10.5 mg of medication in tablet form. Each tablet contained 3.5 mg of medication. How many tablets were given to the patient?
7. A serving of meat weighs 0.3 lb. How many servings are in a large piece of meat weighing 12.6 lb?

8. There are 47 residents at an assisted-living facility. If four attendants are on duty during evening hours, for how many residents is each attendant responsible? (Round to the nearest whole number.)
9. A hospital charged $437.50 for five laborary tests. How much did the hospital charge for one test? (Assume that all tests cost the same.)
10. A bottle contains 35 tablets of medication. If a dosage consists of two tablets, how many complete dosages are in the bottle? (Ignore a partial dose.)
11. A bottle contains 57 mL of vaccine. If the dosage of vaccine is 1.2 mL, how many complete dosages are in the bottle? (Ignore a partial dose.)
12. If five nurses split a $19.50 bill for pizza, what is each nurse's share?

EXERCISES IN MIXED APPLICATIONS

(*Answers are on pages 112–113.*)

Solve these application problems using addition, subtraction, multiplication, and/or division. Some problems may require multiple steps.

1. A patient's bill for a doctor's visit was $89.65. The prescription cost $35.87. What was the total cost for the patient?
2. A container holds 34 mL of an experimental drug. How many 1.6 mL doses can be administered from the container?
3. A patient weighed 90.7 kg before beginning a weight reduction program. At the end of three months, the patient weighed 87.6 kg. How much weight did the patient lose.
4. How many 0.16 fl oz doses of cough syrup are in a bottle containing 4.4 fl oz?
5. The doctor prescribed 1.5 tablets to be given to a patient three times a day for 14 days. How many tablets were prescribed?
6. A doctor ordered 15 mg of medication for a patient. The nurse misread the order and gave the patient 1.5 mg of medication. How much more medication should the patient be given to meet the doctor's order?
7. A new nurse reported a patient's temperature as 37.25°C. The nurse in charge told the new nurse to round this temperature to the nearest degree. What was the rounded temperature?

8. A bottle contains 32.4 fl oz of medication. How many 0.4 fl oz doses will this bottle provide?
9. A doctor ordered 35 mg of medication for a patient. The nurse misread the order and gave the patient 3.5 mg of medication. How much more medication should the patient be given to meet the doctor's order?
10. A medical lab charges $162.75 for a laboratory test. If seven tests are done, what are the total lab charges?
11. A critical-care patient must be monitored constantly. If 16 nurses share this duty evenly, how many hours a week will each nurse be with this patient? (There are 24 hours in a day and 7 days in a week.)
12. Ella May earned $113.10 for 3.25 hours of nursing. Ella June earned $102.05 for the same 3.25 hours of nursing. Compared to Ella June, how much more per hour is Ella May paid?

SECTION TEST: DIVIDING DECIMALS

(Answers are on page 114.)

Divide these numbers.

1. $2.64 \div 2$
2. $63.99 \div 3$
3. $0.153 \div 5$
4. $18.6 \div 0.6$
5. $0.3647 \div 0.07$
6. $0.91 \div 0.008$
7. $1.368 \div 4.5$
8. $35.035 \div 0.5$

Divide these numbers, showing the remainders as fractions.

9. $12.3 \div 0.5$
10. $11.7 \div 0.8$

Divide these numbers, showing the remainders as decimals.

11. $5.5 \div 8.8$
12. $1.44 \div 1.6$

13. *Round this answer to the nearest tenth:* $0.959 \div 0.7$.

14. *Round this answer to the nearest hundredth:* $6 \div 11$.

Divide these numbers by the power of 10 indicated.

15. $34.58 \div 10$
16. $86.51 \div 100$
17. $19.46 \div 1000$
18. $2 \div 10$

19. A nurse earns $1262 for 40 hours of work before deductions and taxes. How much does he make an hour?

20. A nurse earns $1103.25 for 37.5 hours of work before deductions and taxes. How much does she make an hour?

21. A clinic received a delivery of 500 mL of vaccine. If each dosage is 2.5 mL, how many doses of vaccine will this delivery yield?

22. A doctor has ordered a 2000-calorie diet for a patient. If the calories are spread evenly between three meals, how many calories will the patient be allowed to have at each meal? (Round to the nearest whole calorie.)

23. A patient, thankful for the wonderful care she received during her recovery, left a $175 check to be split evenly among her four nurses. How much did each nurse receive?

24. A patient received a total of 13.5 mg of medication from nine tablets. What is the strength of each tablet?

ANSWERS TO EXERCISES IN DIVIDING DECIMALS BY WHOLE NUMBERS

(Exercises are on page 86.)

1. 43.7
2. 3.213
3. 2.12
4. 6.8
5. 7.6
6. 5.19
7. 4.3
8. 3.2
9. 2.3

ANSWERS TO EXERCISES IN DIVIDING A NUMBER BY A DECIMAL

(Exercises are on page 90.)

1. 15
2. 16
3. 83
4. 1.5
5. 11.3
6. 6.4
7. 0.82
8. 3.2
9. 14

ANSWERS TO EXERCISES IN DIVIDING WITH ZEROS IN THE QUOTIENT

(Exercises are on page 93.)

1. 2.03
2. 80.7
3. 1.0203
4. 9.009
5. 3.008
6. 6.006

ANSWERS TO EXERCISES IN DIVIDING WITH REMAINDERS

(Exercises are on page 96.)

1. $3\frac{1}{5}$
2. $3\frac{5}{17}$
3. $1\frac{1}{6}$
4. $4\frac{3}{4}$
5. $8\frac{2}{11}$
6. $2\frac{19}{21}$
7. 0.75
8. 0.375
9. 0.875
10. 0.1875
11. 0.5625
12. 0.34375

ANSWERS TO EXERCISES IN DIVIDING TO A FIXED PLACE ACCURACY

(Exercises are on page 100.)

1. 1.14, which rounds to 1.1
2. 0.88, which rounds to 0.9
3. 2.66, which rounds to 2.7
4. 0.555, which rounds to 0.56
5. 0.714, which rounds to 0.71
6. 0.454, which rounds to 0.45

7. 0.6363, which rounds to 0.636
8. 0.7777, which rounds to 0.778
9. 0.5384, which rounds to 0.538

ANSWERS TO EXERCISES IN DIVIDING BY A POWER OF 10

(Exercises are on page 102.)

1. 6.83	2. 0.8	3. 0.04
4. 1.28	5. 0.128	6. 0.0017
7. 0.9572	8. 0.0016	9. 0.005

ANSWERS TO EXERCISES IN DIVISION APPLICATIONS

(Exercises are on pages 104–105.)

1. Divide the amount of time (4.5 hours) by the length of time it takes to examine one patient (0.25 hours) to find the number of patients the doctor can examine in 4.5 hours: $4.5 \div 0.25 = 18$. The doctor can examine 18 patients in 4.5 hours.

2. Solve this problem the same way the previous problem was solved. Divide the amount of time (4.5 hours) by the length of time it takes to examine one patient (0.75 hours) to find the number of patients the doctor can examine in 4.5 hours: $4.5 \div 0.75 = 6$. This doctor can examine six patients in 4.5 hours.

3. Divide the amount the bottle holds (120 mL) by the amount of one dose (1.5 mL) to find the number of doses of medication in the bottle: $120 \div 1.5 = 80$. There are 80 doses in the bottle.

4. This problem is similar to the previous one and is solved the same way. Divide the amount of disinfectant (67.5 mL) by the amount needed for each batch (4 mL) to find the number of batches of cleaning solution that can be made from a 67.5 mL container: $67.5 \div 4 = 16.875$. Because there is enough to make 16 full batches with 0.875 mL of disinfectant left over, this amount of disinfectant can make 16 complete batches of cleaning solution. The amount of disinfectant left over (0.875 mL) is ignored.

5. Divide the 24-hour time period by 5 to find how many hours each nurse must monitor the patient: $24 \div 5 = 4.8$. Each nurse must monitor the patient 4.8 hours.

6. Divide the total medication given (10.5 mg) by the amount each tablet contains (3.5 mg) to find how many tablets were given: $10.5 \div 3.5 = 3$. Three tablets were given to the patient.

7. Divide the total amount of meat (12.6 lb) by the amount of each serving (0.3 lb) to find the number of servings in 12.6 lb of meat: $12.6 \div 0.3 = 42$. There are 42 servings in the large piece of meat.

8. Divide the number of residents (47) by the number of attendants (4) to find the number of residents for which each attendant is responsible: $47 \div 4 = 11.75$, which rounds to 12. Each attendant is responsible for 12 residents.

9. Divide the total amount charged ($437.50) by the number of tests (5) to find the charge for one test: $\$437.50 \div 5 = \$87.50$. The hospital charges $87.50 for one test.

10. Divide the number of tablets in the bottle (35) by the number of tablets in a dosage (2) to find the number of dosages in the bottle: $35 \div 2 = 17.5$. There are 17 complete dosages in the bottle. The partial dosage (0.5) is ignored.

11. Divide the amount of vaccine in the bottle (57 mL) by the amount of vaccine in a dosage (1.2 mL) to find the number of dosages in the bottle: $57 \div 1.2 = 47.5$. There are 47 complete dosages in the bottle. The partial dosage (0.5) is ignored.

12. Divide the bill for pizza ($19.50) by the number of nurses (5) to find each nurse's share: $19.50 \div 5 = 3.9$. Each nurse's share is $3.90.

ANSWERS TO EXERCISES IN MIXED APPLICATIONS

(Exercises are on pages 106–107.)

1. This is an addition problem. Add the patient's bill ($89.65) and the cost of the prescription ($35.87) to find the total cost for the patient: $89.65 + 35.87 = 125.52$. The total cost for the patient was $125.52.

2. This is a division problem. Divide the amount the container holds (34 mL) by the amount of one dose (1.6 mL) to find the total number of doses in the container: $34 \div 1.6 = 21.25$. Because a partial dose would not be given, 21 doses can be administered from the container.

3. This is a subtraction problem. Subtract the starting weight (90.7 kg) from the current weight (87.6 kg) to find the amount of weight the patient lost: $90.7 - 87.6 = 3.1$. The patient lost 3.1 kg.

4. This is a division problem. Divide the total amount in the bottle (4.4 fl oz) by the amount of one dose (0.16 fl oz) to find the number of doses in the bottle: $4.4 \div 0.16 = 27.5$. Because a partial dose would not be given, there are 27 doses of cough syrup in the bottle.

5. This is a multistep multiplication problem. Multiply the number of tablets (1.5) times the number of times the tablets were given in one day (3) to find the total number of tablets given in one day: $1.5 \times 3 = 4.5$. Therefore, 4.5 tablets were given in one day.

   Now multiply the number of tablets given in one day times the number of days (14 days) to find the number of tablets prescribed in 14 days: $4.5 \times 14 = 63$. So 63 tablets were prescribed.

6. This is a subtraction problem. Subtract the amount of medication the nurse gave the patient (1.5 mg) from the amount of medication the doctor ordered (15 mg) to find the amount of medication the patient still needs: $15 - 1.5 = 13.5$. The patient should be given an additional 13.5 mg of medication to meet the doctor's order.

7. Rounding 37.25°C to the nearest whole degree requires knowledge of place value. The digit 7 is in the units place. Because the digit to its right is 2 (which is not 5 or larger), the digits to the right of the decimal point are dropped. 37.25°C rounded to the nearest whole degree is 37°C.

8. This is a division problem. Divide the total amount in the bottle (32.4 fl oz) by the amount of one dose (0.4 fl oz) to find the number of doses in the bottle: $32.4 \div 0.4 = 81$. This bottle will provide 81 doses.

9. This is a subtraction problem. Subtract the amount the nurse gave (3.5 mg) from the amount the doctor ordered (35 mg) to find how much more medication the patient needs: $35 - 3.5 = 31.5$. The patient should be given an additional 31.5 mg to meet the doctor's order.

10. This is a mutliplication problem. Multiply the charge for one test ($162.75) times the number of tests (7) to find the total lab charges: $162.75 \times 7 = 1139.25$. The total lab charges are $1139.25.

11. This is a multistep problem. First, find how many hours the patient needs to be monitored. Multiply the hours in a day (24 hours) times the number of days (7 days): $24 \times 7 = 168$. The patient needs to be monitored a total of 168 hours.

    Next, divide the number of hours of monitoring (168 hours) by the number of nurses (16) to find how many hours each nurse must monitor the patient: $168 \div 16 = 10.5$. Each nurse will be with the patient 10.5 hours a week.

12. This is a multistep problem. First, calculate Ella May's rate of pay by dividing her pay ($113.10) by the number of hours she worked (3.25): $113.10 \div 3.25 = 34.80$. Ella May's rate of pay is $34.80.

    Next, calculate Ella June's rate of pay by dividing her pay ($102.05) by the number of hours she worked (3.25): $102.05 \div 3.25 = 31.40$. Ella June's rate of pay is $31.40.

    Finally, subtract Ella June's rate of pay ($31.40) from Ella May's rate of pay ($34.80) to find how much more Ella May is paid: $34.80 – $31.40 = $3.40. Ella May is paid $3.40 more per hour.

ANSWERS TO SECTION TEST: DIVIDING DECIMALS

(Section Test is on pages 108–109.)

1. 1.32
2. 21.33
3. 0.0306
4. 31
5. 5.21
6. 113.75
7. 0.304
8. 70.07
9. $24\frac{3}{5}$
10. $14\frac{5}{8}$
11. 0.625
12. 0.9
13. 1.37, which rounds to 1.4
14. 0.545, which rounds to 0.55
15. 3.458
16. 0.8651
17. 0.01945
18. 0.2
19. Divide the nurse's earnings ($1262) by the number of hours he works (40) to find how much he makes an hour: $1262 \div 40 = 31.55$. He makes $31.55 an hour.
20. Divide the nurse's earnings ($1103.25) by the number of hours she works (37.5) to find how much she makes an hour: $1103.25 \div 37.5 = 29.42$. She makes $29.42 an hour.
21. Divide the amount of vaccine (500 mL) by the amount in each dose (2.5 mL) to find the number of doses in this amount of vaccine: $500 \div 2.5 = 200$. This delivery will yield 200 doses.
22. Divide the total number of calories (2000) by the number of meals (3) to find the number of calories for each meal: $2000 \div 3 = 666.6$. The answer rounds to 667. The patient will be allowed to have 667 calories at each meal.
23. Divide the amount of the check ($175) by the number of nurses (4) to find how much each nurse received: $175 \div 4 = 43.75$. Each nurse received $43.75.
24. Divide the number of milligrams (13.5 mg) by the number of tablets (9) to find the strength of each tablet: $13.5 \div 9 = 1.5$. The strength of each tablet is 1.5 mg.

Locating Decimal Points

The **decimal point** appears just to the right of the units (also called ones) place value and separates the whole number portion from the decimal portion of the number. Every number has a decimal point, yet it may not always be visible. When a decimal point is not needed, it usually is not shown. If the decimal point is not visible in a number, it is located just to the right of the last digit in the number.

Determining Place Value

Compare these two amounts of money: $543.21 and $123.45. The first amount represents more money. Notice that each amount has a dollar sign, a decimal point, and the same digits 1 through 5, yet the amounts are different because of how the digits are positioned. The position of a digit in relationship to the digits around it is called **place value.**

The Place Value Chart

The place value chart is shown in Figure S-1.

←Number gets larger Number gets smaller→

Whole Numbers								Decimal Numbers					
Millions	Hundred Thousands	Ten Thousands	Thousands	Hundreds	Tens	Units or Ones	Decimal Point	Tenths	Hundredths	Thousandths	Ten-thousandths	Hundred-thousandths	Millionths

Figure S-1

Consider the following facts about decimals:

- In reading a number, the decimal point is read as *and*. The word *and* is not said anywhere else in the number.
- Numbers to the right of the decimal point are smaller than 1, and numbers to the left of the decimal point are whole numbers.
- Starting from the decimal point and moving to the left in the whole number portion, a comma is used to separate groups of three digits.
- No commas are used to the right of the decimal point.
- All decimal places end with the letters *ths.*
- All of the decimal place values have a corresponding whole number place value.
- There is no corresponding decimal position for the units position.
- The decimal places of ten-thousandths and hundred-thousandths use a hyphen, while ten thousands and hundred thousands places do not.
- If there is no whole number with the decimal, place a zero in the units place.

Reading Decimal Numbers

To read a number that has a decimal in it, first read the whole number part of the number. Be sure to say the grouping name (for example, thousand or million). The decimal point is read as *and.* Next, read the decimal part of the number as if it were a whole number. Then say the name of the place value that is farthest to the right. The number 1.234 would be read as *one and two hundred thirty-four thousandths.*

Writing Decimal Numbers in Digits

To write a number in digits that has a decimal in it, first write the digits of the whole number portion. Next, place the decimal point. Finally, write the decimal portion of the number. If necessary, use zeros to maintain proper place value.

- Use *and* only to represent the decimal point.
- Use a hyphen between the numbers 21 to 99 no matter where they appear in the number.
- Use commas to separate the groups of numbers in whole numbers.
- Do not use commas to separate groups of numbers in decimals as you would in whole numbers.

Identifying Necessary and Unnecessary Zeros

When there is no whole number with a decimal, place a zero in the units place value; this is the leading zero. Its purpose is to help identify the location of the decimal point. There should be only one leading zero.

Zeros may be added to the right of the last nonzero digit of a decimal without changing the value of the number. When the number is given as an answer, these zeros are usually discarded. An exception is made in the case of money. For example, $0.50 is not changed to $0.5.

Calculators generally remove unnecessary zeros at the end of a decimal number. Calculators may also add a zero in the units place when there are no whole numbers.

Comparing Decimals

To compare two decimal numbers, first determine the smallest place value of the decimals. Add enough zeros to the other number so that both numbers have the same place values. Then compare the two numbers.

Rounding to a Specific Place Value

Step 1: Locate the digit in the specific place value to be rounded. This is the **rounding digit.** You may find that underlining it is helpful.

Step 2: Look at the digit directly to its right. If this digit is 5 or larger, increase the rounding digit by one. If this digit is not 5 or larger, do not change the rounding digit.

Step 3: For places to the right of the decimal point, drop all digits after the rounded digit. If the number represents money, zeros may be added to give two decimal places.

Lining Up Decimals in Addition

The addition of decimals is identical to the addition of whole numbers. Lining up the decimal points ensures that the place values are positioned properly. If a decimal does not appear in a number, the decimal point is immediately after the last digit.

Adding Zeros in Addition

It is often necessary to add extra zeros to indicate empty place values on the decimal side of the number. This helps keep the numbers lined up and visually assists in addition.

Adding Decimals

When adding numbers with decimals in them, start the addition with the column that has the smallest place value. This is the column at the right. Continue to add columns, moving toward the left until all columns are added. The numbers being added are called **addends,** and the answer is called the **sum.**

Carrying in Addition

When the sum of the digits for a place value is larger than 9, part of the number is carried to the next place value. For example, $5 + 8 = 13$. For the number 13, the 1 represents a ten because it is in the tens place value and the 3 represents 3 units ($10 + 3 = 13$). The digit 3 remains in the units place, and the digit 1 is carried to the tens place.

Solving Addition Applications

Step 1: Read the problem carefully. Pay close attention to the numbers in the problem.

Step 2: Read the question carefully. What exactly is it looking for? What labels will be used in the answer?

Step 3: Eliminate any unnecessary information.

Step 4: Draw a diagram if it is helpful.

Step 5: Decide how to solve the problem. Some problems may require more than one step.

Step 6: Round the numbers to the highest place value and estimate the answer.

Step 7: Calculate the final answer and compare it with the estimate.

Step 8: Include the label in the answer.

Adding versus Subtracting

Subtraction is often called the opposite of addition. When one number is added to another, the answer is the **sum.** When one of the numbers is subtracted from the sum, the other number is the **difference.**

Avoiding Common Mistakes in Adding and Subtracting Decimals

- Lining up the place values of the numbers improperly
- Using sloppy handwriting or sloppy positioning of the numbers
- Copying the numbers incorrectly
- Carrying improperly
- Using incorrect math facts

Setting Up a Subtraction Problem

The same rules used for addition apply to subtraction: line up the decimal points in the numbers and add zeros if necessary. Sometimes the way a problem is worded can be confusing. It is important to know which number is the starting point (the top number in a subtraction problem). If the problem is worded *subtract 12 from 36,* 36 is the starting number. Thus, it is on top. On the other hand, if the problem is worded *40 minus 18,* 40 is the starting number.

Subtracting without Borrowing

As in addition, begin subtracting with the smallest place value. This is the place value farthest to the right. Continue subtracting each place value in order from right to left.

Checking a Subtraction Problem

Because addition is the opposite of subtraction, addition is used to check the answer to a subtraction problem. Add the answer to the number being subtracted; the result will be the top number.

Subtracting with Borrowing

In addition, when an amount is larger than 9, part of it is **carried** to the next place value. In subtraction, there is an opposite process called **borrowing.** An amount is removed from a larger place value, and its equivalent is added to the smaller place value.

Working with Zeros When Borrowing

When borrowing, if a zero is in the next column, it is necessary to borrow from the next nonzero column. When there is more than one zero, continue to the next nonzero column to borrow.

Solving Subtraction Applications

Use subtraction to answer questions that ask for the difference between two numbers. The following key words may indicate the need to subtract: *how much greater than; how much less than; how much of an increase or decrease; how many more;* and *how much farther, bigger, smaller, or heavier.* For the subtraction process, a smaller amount is generally removed from an overall amount.

Multiplication Concepts

When multiplying numbers, it does not matter which number is on the top and which is on the bottom. The answer will be the same. Generally, the number with the fewest digits is on the bottom to make the multiplication easier.

The major difference between the process of multiplication of decimals and the process of addition and subtraction of decimals is that in multiplication, the decimal points are *not* lined up. The numbers to be multiplied are written without regard to their place value. After the numbers are multiplied, the decimal point is positioned in the answer.

Positioning the Decimal Point in an Answer

The position of the decimal point in an answer is determined once the numbers are multiplied. First, count the number of places to the right of the decimal points in both numbers. Second, starting from the far right place value, move the decimal point in the answer the same number of places to the left. If no decimal appears in a number, the decimal is assumed to be just to the right of the last digit.

If there are not enough decimal places in the answer to reposition the decimal point, additional zeros may need to be added. If the decimal point appears before the first nonzero digit, be sure to add a leading zero.

Multiplying a Number Times a Number

To multiply a number times another number, position the numbers for multiplication. Then multiply the first digit in the second number times all of the digits in the first number and record the answer below the line. This is the first line of the answer.

If the multiplying number has more than one digit, multiply by the second digit in the second number. Because the second digit is actually in the tens place, put a zero in the units place in the second line of the answer. This preserves proper place value. Then multiply the second digit times all of the numbers in the top number and record the answer on the second answer line.

If there is a third digit to be multiplied, place two zeros on the third answer line because the third digit is actually in the hundreds place. Continue multiplying as before. (Subsequent digits are handled in the same manner.)

When all of the digits have been multiplied, add all of the lines of the answer to get the final answer. Finally, position the decimal point properly.

Carrying in Multiplication

In the process of multiplying, if two numbers multiplied together result in an answer that is larger than 9, part of the answer needs to be carried to the next place value. This is similar to the carrying explained in Section 2: Addition of Decimals.

Working with Zeros in Multiplication

Working with zeros sometimes causes confusion in the multiplication process. The zeros are necessary in the numbers because they ensure that the digits are in their proper place. There is a big difference between $12, $102, and $1002.

Do not ignore the zeros. Multiply with the zeros even though zero times any number is zero. Remember that the use of the zero is necessary to put the digits in their proper place value.

Solving Multiplication Applications

Multiplication application problems generally provide information about one item and ask for information representing several items. For instance, if one shirt costs $5, how much would three shirts cost? To solve this problem, multiply the cost of one shirt ($5) by the number of shirts (3) to get the cost of three shirts ($15).

Division Concepts

Division of decimals is similar to division of whole numbers. The only real difference is the positioning of the decimal point in the answer. The number being divided is called the **dividend.** The number being divided into the dividend is called the **divisor.** The answer is the **quotient.** When a divisor does not divide evenly into the dividend, the leftover part is called a **remainder.**

Figure S-2 shows the location of these terms in a division problem.

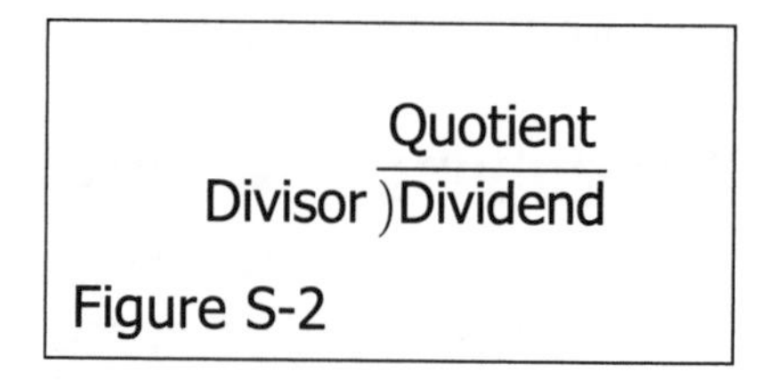

Figure S-2

When dividing a decimal by a whole number, simply position the decimal point in the answer (quotient) above the decimal point in the number being divided (dividend).

Positioning the Decimal Point in Division

When a number is divided by a decimal, the decimal must be removed from the divisor. First, move the decimal point to the position just after the last digit in the divisor. Then discard any leading zeros in the divisor. Finally, move the decimal in the dividend the same number of places to the right as was done with the divisor. Add zeros to create decimal places if necessary. Place the decimal point in the quotient (answer) directly above the decimal point in the dividend. It is important to move the decimal point the same number of places in both the divisor and the dividend.

Quotients with Zeros in the Middle

If the number being divided is smaller than the divisor, it will go zero times. The zero is placed in the quotient to preserve the proper place value in the answer. Then it is necessary to bring down the next number from the dividend to get a number large enough to be divided by the divisor.

Quotients with Zeros at the End

A common error in division involves zeros at the end of the quotient. In some division problems, all nonzero digits in the dividend may be divided, yet zeros remain in the dividend. To maintain proper place value, it is necessary to complete the division process to get zeros in the quotient. The mistake some students make is stopping the division process too soon.

Working with Remainders

A **remainder** occurs when the divisor does not divide evenly into the dividend. Following are three methods of dealing with remainders:

- Show the remainder as a fraction, with the remainder as the numerator and the divisor as the denominator. Reduce the fraction if possible. To avoid having a decimal and a fraction in the same number, stop dividing before a decimal is in the quotient.
- Add zeros to the dividend and continue the division until there is no remainder.
- Round to a specific place value. This method is applicable to the healthcare professional who frequently rounds to the nearest tenth or hundredth.

Dividing to a Fixed Place Accuracy

Healthcare professionals often work with medications that are rounded to the nearest tenth or hundredth. Dividing to a specific place value is called **dividing to a fixed place accuracy.**

To divide to a fixed place accuracy, follow these steps:

Step 1: Determine how many places will be needed after the decimal point in the answer.

Step 2: Add one more place value (for rounding purposes).

Step 3: Do the division. Ignore any remainder.

Step 4: Locate the digit in the specific place value to be rounded. This is the rounding digit.

Step 5A: Look at the digit directly to its right. If this digit is 5 or larger, increase the rounding digit by one.

Step 5B: If this digit is not 5 or larger, do not change the rounding digit. Drop all digits to the right of the rounding digit.

Dividing by a Power of 10

A power of 10 is any number whose first digit is 1 and the remaining digits are zeros. These numbers are powers of 10: 10, 100, 1000, 10,000, etc.

To divide by a power of 10, count the number of zeros in the power of 10. Then move the decimal point to the left the same number of places. When a number is divided by a power of 10, the answer is smaller than the dividend. Moving the decimal point to the left results in a smaller answer. It may be necessary to add leading zeros.

Thus, to divide 12.34 by 10, move the decimal point one place to the left so that the number becomes 1.234. To divide that same number by 100, move the decimal point two places to the left so that the number becomes 0.1234. To divide the same number by 1000, move the decimal point three places to the left so that the number becomes 0.01234.

Solving Division Applications

Division takes a larger quantity and divides it into an equal number of smaller parts. For example, if $20 is being evenly divided among five children, $20 would be divided by 5 to get an answer of $4. Thus, each child would get $4. To verify that this is correct, if the $4 from each child were added together, there would be $20 ($4 × 5 = $20).

Cumulative Test on Decimals

(Answers are on pages 130–134.)

1. Where is the decimal point in a number when the decimal point is not showing?

2. When reading a number that has decimals in it, what word is used to represent the decimal point?

3. Where might commas be used in a number that includes a decimal, to the right or the left of the decimal point?

4. If a decimal does not include a whole number, what digit is placed in the units place value?

5. Are numbers to the right of the decimal point smaller or larger than 1?

Use the number 12,345.6789 *to answer the following questions.*

6. Which digit is in the hundredths position?

7. Which digit is in the thousands position?

8. Which digit is in the ten-thousandths position?

9. Which digit is in the units position?

10. Which digit is in the tenths position?

Write these words as digits.

11. fifty-six and fifty-seven hundredths

12. six and five tenths

13. eight thousandths

14. thirty-four thousand and thirty-four ten-thousandths

Rewrite these decimals by supplying necessary zeros or eliminating unnecessary zeros.

15. .13

16. 1.300

17. 00.01300

Put these decimals in order from smallest to largest.

18. 0.46, 0.064, 0.64, 0.046

Round these decimals to the nearest whole number.

19. 2.38

20. 2.83

Round these decimals to the nearest tenth.

21. 7.94

22. 7.95

Add these numbers.

23. 4.21 and 3.65

24. 6.48 and 0.095

25. 6.387, 25.7, and 1.875

26. 0.06, 0.73, and 0.21

Subtract these numbers.

27. Subtract 2.1 from 3.8

28. 0.2 minus 0.08

29. $\begin{array}{r} 5.0 \\ -\ 1.8 \\ \hline \end{array}$

30. $\begin{array}{r} 2.15 \\ -\ 0.78 \\ \hline \end{array}$

31. $\begin{array}{r} 0.403 \\ -\ 0.094 \\ \hline \end{array}$

Multiply these numbers.

32. $\begin{array}{r} 3.84 \\ \times\ 0.5 \\ \hline \end{array}$

33. $\begin{array}{r} 23.4 \\ \times\ 2.34 \\ \hline \end{array}$

34. $\begin{array}{r} 0.0625 \\ \times\ 0.0375 \\ \hline \end{array}$

35. $\begin{array}{r} 1.06 \\ \times\ 0.05 \\ \hline \end{array}$

36. $\begin{array}{r} 0.608 \\ \times\ 0.205 \\ \hline \end{array}$

37. $\begin{array}{r} 2.02 \\ \times\ 0.505 \\ \hline \end{array}$

Divide these numbers.

38. Divide 46.28 by 2

39. Divide 4.628 by 0.02

40. Divide 5 by 0.8

41. Divide 0.14 by 1.6

42. Divide 1.025 by 0.5

43. Divide 14.07 by 0.7

44. Divide 10.01667 by 0.3

45. Divide 1 by 0.08

Show the remainders as indicated.

46. Show the answer as a whole number with a fraction: $1.6 \div 0.5$

47. Show the answer as a decimal: $0.3 \div 8$

48. Round the answer to the nearest tenth: $9 \div 1.1$

49. Round the answer to the nearest hundredth: $2 \div 3$

50. Round the answer to the nearest thousandth: $0.6 \div 0.11$

Solve these application problems using addition, subtraction, multiplication, and division. Some of these problems are multistep.

51. If a nurse is paid $38.75 an hour, how much will she earn in 8 hours?

52. A patient received 2.5 mL of medication on Monday, 1.75 mL on Tuesday, and 2.25 mL on Wednesday. How much medication did the patient receive?

53. If a nurse earns $174.35 in 5.5 hours, how much is the nurse paid an hour?

54. A patient is supposed to drink 8 oz of orange juice a day. If the patient already drank 5.5 oz, how much more orange juice does he need to drink?

55. Nurses' aides are required to work 37.5 hours a week. How many hours will seven nurses' aides work in one week?

56. One patient weighs 79.8 kg, and her sister weighs 82.4 kg. How much more does the patient's sister weigh?

57. A doctor ordered 25 mg of medication for a patient. The nurse misread the instructions and gave the patient 2.5 mg. How much more medication does the patient need?

58. An 8 oz bottle of a name brand cold remedy sells for $17.99. A drug store sells a 4 oz generic brand for $5.99. If a cold sufferer buys 16 oz of medication, which is the better deal—the name brand or the generic brand? By how much is it a better buy?

59. There are four open bottles of the same cough syrup in a medicine cabinet. One bottle contains 3.25 mL, another contains 0.75 mL, a third contains 2 mL, and the fourth contains 1.75 mL. How many milliliters of cough syrup are there?

60. A patient's fluid output was measured over a 24-hour period as 0.2 L, 0.125 L, 0.08 L, and 0.14 L. What was the patient's total fluid output?

61. How much medication is needed if 2.3 mL injections are administered to 31 patients?

62. If the correct dosage for a particular medication is 2.5 mL, how many patients can receive the medication if the total supply is 60 mL?

63. The East Street Clinic administered 26 injections of flu vaccine, and the West Street Clinic administered 31 injections of the same flu vaccine. If each injection is 1.8 mL, what was the total amount of flu vaccine administered at both clinics?

64. A patient's physical therapy costs $86.50 an hour. If a patient receives 0.75 hour of therapy, what is the patient's bill?

65. A patient weighing 92.3 kg lost 3.1 kg over a ten-day period. How much does the patient weigh now?

66. A doctor's visit cost $125.75. The patient paid the insurance co-pay of $20. A bill was sent to the insurance company. What was the amount of the bill?

67. A nurse's aide earned $169.43 for 7.75 hours of work. A supervising nurse earned $108.06 for 3.25 hours of work. How much more an hour is the supervising nurse paid than the nurse's aide? (Round all amounts to the nearest penny.)

68. A container holds 1500 g of medication in powder form. If 15.5 g is needed for treatment, how many treatments will this container provide?

69. If an opened box contains six 7.25 oz bottles of hand sanitizer, and another opened box contains four 7.25 oz bottles of hand sanitizer, how many bottles of hand sanitizer are there?

70. A patient lacking medical coverage for a particular procedure was charged for two X-rays costing \$185.37 each, six bandages costing \$12.81 each, and a splint costing \$17.95. The patient paid \$50 and agreed to pay the rest in five equal payments. What is the amount of each payment?

ANSWERS TO CUMULATIVE TEST ON DECIMALS

1. When the decimal point in a number is not showing, the decimal point is just to the right of the rightmost digit.
2. The word *and* is used to represent the decimal point. This is the only time the word *and* should be used when a number is read.
3. Commas might be used to the left of the decimal point, but they are *never* used to the right of the decimal point.
4. A zero is placed to the left of the decimal point (in the units place) to indicate that there are no whole numbers.
5. Numbers to the right of the decimal point are smaller than 1.
6. The digit 7 is in the hundredths position.
7. The digit 2 is in the thousands position.
8. The digit 9 is in the ten-thousandths position.
9. The digit 5 is in the units position.
10. The digit 6 is in the tenths position.

11. 56.57 12. 6.5 13. 0.008 14. 34,000.0034

15. 0.13 16. 1.3 17. 0.013

18. 0.046, 0.064 0.46, 0.64

19. 2 20. 3 21. 7.9 22. 8

23. $\begin{array}{r} 4.21 \\ +\ 3.65 \\ \hline 7.86 \end{array}$

24. $\begin{array}{r} 6.480 \\ +\ 0.095 \\ \hline 6.575 \end{array}$

25. $\begin{array}{r} 6.387 \\ 25.700 \\ +\ 1.875 \\ \hline 33.962 \end{array}$

26. $\begin{array}{r} 0.06 \\ 0.73 \\ +\ 0.21 \\ \hline 1.00 \end{array}$

answer: 1

27. $\begin{array}{r} 3.8 \\ -\ 2.1 \\ \hline 1.7 \end{array}$

28. $\begin{array}{r} 0.20 \\ -\ 0.08 \\ \hline 0.12 \end{array}$

29. $\begin{array}{r} 5.0 \\ -\ 1.8 \\ \hline 3.2 \end{array}$

30. $\begin{array}{r} 2.15 \\ -\ 0.78 \\ \hline 1.37 \end{array}$

31. $\begin{array}{r} 0.403 \\ -\ 0.094 \\ \hline 0.309 \end{array}$

```
32.   3.84
    × 0.5
     1920
answer: 1.92
```

```
33.     23.4
      × 2.34
         936
        7020
       46800
       54756
answer: 54.756
```

```
34.   0.0625
    × 0.0375
        3125
       43750
      187500
      234375
answer: 0.00234375
```

```
35.   1.06
    × 0.05
       530
answer: 0.053
```

```
36.   0.608
    × 0.205
       3040
      00000
     121600
     124640
answer: 0.12464
```

```
37.     2.02
     × 0.505
        1010
        0000
      101000
      102010
answer: 1.0201
```

38. 23.14
39. 231.4
40. 6.25
41. 0.0875
42. 2.05
43. 20.1
44. 33.3889
45. 12.5

While most of these division problems have not been shown, several involving remainders are provided for clarity.

46. Position the numbers for division. Move the decimal points so that there is no decimal in the divisor. Stop dividing when there is a digit in the units place and a remainder. Create a fraction by placing the remainder (1) as the numerator over the divisor (5) as the denominator.

    Thus, $1.6 \div 0.5 = 3\frac{1}{5}$ (Figure T-1).

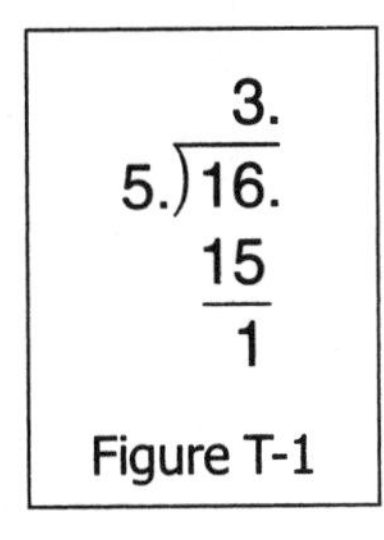

Figure T-1

47. $0.3 \div 8 = 0.0375$

48. Position the numbers for division. Move the decimal points so that there is no decimal in the divisor. Stop dividing once there is a digit in the hundredths place. Rounding 8.18 to the nearest tenth, the answer is 8.2. Thus, $9 \div 1.1 = 8.2$ (Figure T-2).

```
      8.18
11.)90.00
    88
     2 0
     1 1
       90
       88
        2
```

Figure T-2

49. When dividing 2 by 3, add zeros to the right of the decimal place in the dividend. The answer is a repeating number. Stop dividing when there is a digit in the thousandths place. Rounding 0.666 to the nearest hundredth, the answer is 0.67. Thus, 2 ÷ 3 = 0.67 (Figure T-3).

```
     0.666
3.)2.000
   1 8
     20
     18
      20
      18
       2
```

Figure T-3

50. Position the numbers for division. Move the decimal points so there is no decimal in the divisor. Stop dividing when there is a digit in the ten-thousandths place. The answer is a repeating number. Rounding 5.4545 to the nearest thousandth, the answer is 5.455. Thus, 0.6 ÷ 0.11 = 5.455 (Figure T-4).

```
       5.4545
11.)60.0000
    55
     5 0
     4 4
       60
       55
        50
        44
         60
         55
          5
```

Figure T-4

51. This is a multiplication problem. Multiply the pay for one hour ($38.75) times the hours worked (8): $38.75 × 8 = $310.

52. This is an addition problem. Add the three amounts of medication to find the total amount the patient received: 2.5 mL + 1.75 mL + 2.25 mL = 6.5 mL. The patient received 6.5 mL of medication.

53. This is a division problem. Divide the total earnings ($174.35) by the number of hours (5.5) to find how much the nurse is paid an hour: $174.35 ÷ 5.5 = $31.70. The nurse is paid $31.70 an hour.

54. This is a subtraction problem. Subtract what the patient already drank (5.5 oz) from the total amount the patient is supposed to have (8 oz) to find how much more he needs to drink: 8 − 5.5 = 2.5. The patient needs to drink 2.5 more ounces of orange juice.

55. This is a multiplication problem. Multiply the total number of hours nurses' aides are required to work in one week (37.5) times the number of nurses' aides (7) to find the total number of hours they will work in one week: 37.5 × 7 = 262.5. The seven nurses' aides will work 262.5 hours in one week.

56. This is a subtraction problem. Subtract the weight of the patient (79.8 kg) from the weight of her sister (82.4 kg) to find the difference in their weights: 82.4 − 79.8 = 2.6. The patient's sister weighs 2.6 kg more than the patient.

57. This is a subtraction problem. Subtract how much medication the nurse gave the patient (2.5 mg) from how much the doctor ordered (25 mg) to find how much more medication the patient needs: 25 − 2.5 = 22.5. The patient needs 22.5 mg more medication.

58. This is multistep problem that involves multiplication and subtraction. First, calculate how much 16 oz of the name brand medication will cost. Because an 8 oz bottle sells for $17.99, multiply $17.99 by 2 to find the cost of 16 oz: $17.99 × 2 = $35.98.

    Next, calculate how much 16 oz of the generic brand will cost. Because a 4 oz bottle sells for $5.99, multiply $5.99 by 4 to find the cost of 16 oz: $5.99 × 4 = $23.96.

    Because 16 oz of the generic brand sells for $23.96 and 16 oz of the name brand sells for $35.98, the generic brand is cheaper.
    Now subtract the cost of 16 oz of the generic brand from 16 oz of the name brand to find the difference in price: $35.98 − $23.96 = $12.02. The generic brand is cheaper by $12.02.

59. This is an addition problem. Add the contents of the four bottles to find the total amount of cough syrup (Figure T-5). There are 7.75 mL of cough syrup.

$$\begin{array}{r} 3.25 \\ 0.75 \\ 2.00 \\ +1.75 \\ \hline 7.75 \end{array}$$

Figure T-5

60. This is an addition problem. Add the measured fluid output to find the total output (Figure T-6). Be sure to line up the decimal points. The patient's total fluid output was 0.545 L.

$$\begin{array}{r} 0.200 \\ 0.125 \\ 0.080 \\ +\ 0.140 \\ \hline 0.545 \end{array}$$

Figure T-6

61. This is a multiplication problem. Multiply the amount of medication needed for one injection (2.3 mL) times the number of injections (31) to find the total amount of medication needed: $2.3 \times 31 = 71.3$. The amount of medication needed is 71.3 mL.

62. This is a division problem. Divide the total supply (60 mL) by the amount needed for one dosage (2.5 mL) to find the total number of patients that can receive the medication: $60 \div 2.5 = 24$. There are 24 patients who can receive the medication.

63. This is a multistep problem. First, calculate how much flu vaccine was administered at the East Street Clinic. Multiply the amount of each injection (1.8 mL) times the number of injections (26) to find the total amount administered: $1.8 \times 26 = 46.8$. The total amount administered at the East Street Clinic was 46.8 mL.

    Next, calculate how much flu vaccine was administered at the West Street Clinic. Multiply the amount of each injection (1.8 mL) times the number of injections (31) to find the total amount administered: $1.8 \times 31 = 55.8$. The total amount administered at the West Street Clinic was 55.8 mL.

    Now add the amounts administered at the East Street Clinic and the West Street Clinic to find the combined amount: 46.8 mL + 55.8 mL = 102.6 mL. The total amount of flu vaccine administered at both clinics was 102.6 mL.

64. This is a multiplication problem. Multiply the cost of the therapy per hour ($86.50) times the number of hours (0.75) to find the patient's bill: $86.50 × 0.75 = $64.875. Because the answer is referring to money, it should be rounded to the nearest hundredth: $64.875 becomes $64.88. The patient's bill is $64.88.

65. This is a subtraction problem. Subtract the amount the patient lost (3.1 kg) from the patient's original weight (92.3 kg) to find the patient's current weight. Ignore the ten-day period because that is not needed to solve the problem: $92.3 - 3.1 = 89.2$. The patient now weighs 89.2 kg.

66. This is a subtraction problem. Subtract the co-pay ($20) from the cost of the doctor's visit ($125.75) to find the amount of the bill sent to the insurance company: $125.75 − $20.00 = $105.75. The amount of the bill was $105.75.

67. This is a multistep problem. First, calculate how much the nurse's aide earns an hour by dividing the amount earned ($169.43) by the number of hours worked (7.75): $169.43 ÷ 7.75 = $21.862, which rounds to $21.86. The nurse's aide is paid $21.86 an hour.

    Next, calculate how much the supervising nurse earns an hour. Divide the amount earned ($108.06) by the number of hours worked (3.25): $108.06 ÷ 3.25 = $33.249, which rounds to $33.25. The supervising nurse is paid $33.25 an hour.

    Subtract the aide's rate of pay ($21.86) from the supervising nurse's rate of pay ($33.25) to find how much more the supervising nurse is paid: $33.25 − $21.86 = $11.39. The supervising nurse is paid $11.39 more an hour than the nurse's aide.

68. This is a division problem. Divide the contents of the container (1500 g) by the amount needed for each treatment (15.5 g) to find the total number of treatments this container will supply: 1500 ÷ 15.5 = 96.7. Because a partial treatment is not acceptable, the decimal is dropped. This container will provide 96 treatments.

69. This is an addition problem. One box contains six bottles, and the other box contains four bottles. Add 6 + 4 to find 10 bottles of hand sanitizer. The size of the bottles (7.25 oz) is not needed to answer the question.

70. This is a multistep problem. Multiply the cost of the X-rays ($185.37) by the number of X-rays (2) and the cost of the bandages ($12.81) by the number of bandages (6). Add these answers to the cost of the splint to find the total cost: $185.37 × 2 = $370.74 and $12.81 × 6 = $76.86; $370.74 + $76.86 + $17.95 = $465.55. The total cost is $465.55.

    Next, subtract the patient's initial payment ($50) from the total cost of the procedure and supplies ($465.55) to find the amount that needs to be paid: $465.55 − $50.00= $415.55. Finally, divide this number by the total number of equal payments (5) to find the amount of each payment: $415.55 ÷ 5 = $83.11. Each payment is $83.11.

INDEX